Beauty After 40

Beauty After 40

How to Put Time on Your Side

by Susan Sommers

Illustrated by Mary Jo Quay

The Dial Press New York

Published by
The Dial Press
1 Dag Hammarskjold Plaza
New York, New York 10017

Library of Congress Cataloging in Publication Data

Sommers, Susan,
  Beauty after 40.

  Includes index.
  1. Beauty, personal. 2. Middle-aged
women—Health and hygiene. I. Title.
II. Title: Beauty after forty.
RA778.S65   646.7'042   82-2465
ISBN 0-385-27229-4   AACR2

To my mother, with love and appreciation

Acknowledgments

Since so many people gave generously of their time and knowledge to make this book possible, to make this book accurate, I think of it as a joint effort. I gratefully acknowledge the contributions made by all of the experts and celebrities who are quoted herein, and some who are not, like Nancy Durr and Dr. Mannuccio Mannucci.

Special thanks to my editor Nancy van Itallie, my agent Susan Ann Protter, and my very dear and irreplaceable friend Susan Katz, whose help was invaluable, as well as to those who offered much appreciated support and comfort along the way: Louise Sommers, Mary Jo Quay, Stan Place, Dorothy Schefer, Lynn Edlen, Leslie Prager, John Kelley, Emily Rubin, and Ileana Greenwald.

Contents

Part V   For Body and Soul 203

Introduction

Awhile ago, feeling that I was growing older but not necessarily looking better, I decided to try an experiment and practice what I had been preaching as a beauty and health reporter and editor: I vowed to follow a rigorous exercise and revised eating program for three months to see if it would effect a significant change. I had always been the original "Lazy Susan." I occasionally exercised (usually right before I had to put on a bathing suit) and often overindulged. My favorite exercise was lifting fork to mouth. I got away with it because I was naturally slim and wore clothes well. After three months I was so astounded by the change that I kept on going. My skin is clearer (there is some thinking that exercise lessens lining and wrinkling), my posture straighter, I have more energy, and I'm finally sleeping most nights (after years of problems). My body has never been better, nor has my attitude. I feel more confident in all aspects of my life. And I've heard the same story from other women who took action with age—action that's paid off.

In America, especially, age forty has traditionally been approached with trepidation, even loathing, because of the high value society has placed on youth. But happily this outlook is changing. The shift in population toward an older majority has prompted changing ideals. For the women we all want to look as good as are not nymphets. They are in full flower, like Jane Fonda, Ali MacGraw, Sophia Loren—they help to prove that age has only added to their allure. The shift has also prompted ongoing research in the health and beauty sectors, resulting in a host of new products and techniques to meet changing needs.

I wrote *Beauty After 40* to show you how you, too, can be in control of your looks so that you can make your age work for you. All the experts in the beauty and fitness fields tell you about the changes that occur and the best ways of dealing with them. Although it would perhaps be an oversimplification to say that age is simply a state of mind, in many ways it's true. If you explore the options that are available to you throughout life instead of limiting yourself, if you realize that change is inevitable and desirable, in beauty as in everything else, if you recognize that there are as many glorious glamour years after forty as there are before, you can understand the major role that attitude plays. And this book can help you in every way.

Susan Sommers
New York City

Beauty After 40

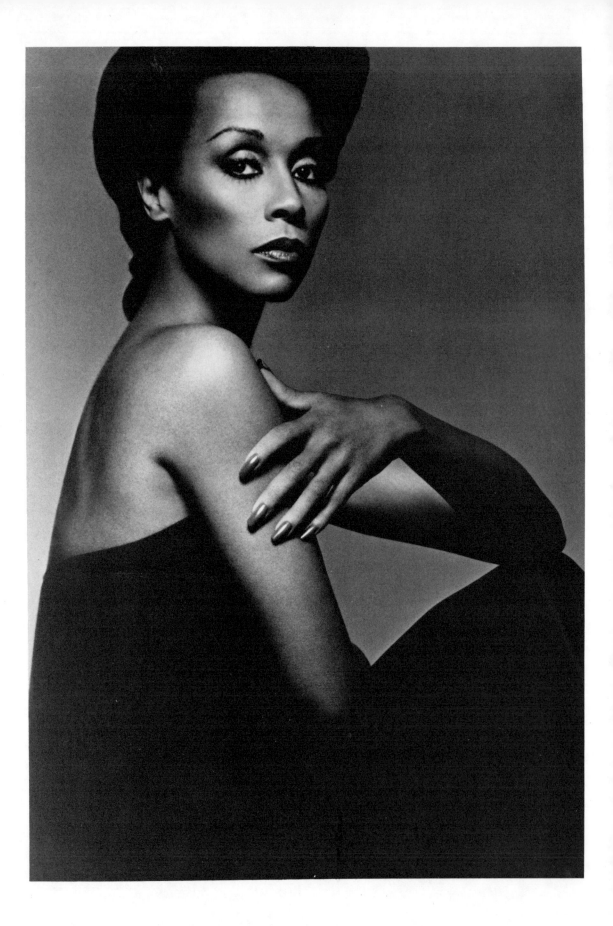

Diahann Carroll

Entertainer

I'm having a marvelous time now. I feel wonderful and I think that this influences how I look more than anything else. I have a greater understanding of who I am and of what makes me comfortable, a very important word.

Socially I find it easier now for women, but this era is a double-edged sword. The freedom is glorious, particularly if you've been of independent character for most of your life, because you don't feel quite so much the outsider as you did when no one else thought like you. Women over forty can relax about being "unmarried," if that is their state. Years ago, it would have been impossible. You were considered a failure when you were not married. Also I don't find the pressures I used to about combining work and family—a combination I always believed in, which was considered foreign in the past.

The cultural stereotype of women over forty is changing, has changed tremendously. Our sexuality has been acknowledged. Before, there was a cutoff point—for example, we could never think of our parents as being sexual. Now we have the freedom of choice. Either you are fortunate enough to recognize and enjoy your sexuality at whatever age, or not. But our culture does place a heavy burden on the man after forty and many men haven't been able to escape this. If a man is convinced that he's supposed to settle down and be "old" because he's just celebrated his fiftieth birthday, it can be frightening. He's fortunate if he can realize that there is no timetable for enjoyment.

I can understand an older woman/younger man relationship, particularly when the woman is busy and not so conventional. A young man can be extremely stimulating. He does not have the cultural and social hang-ups of a man twenty years his senior; he doesn't make the stereotyped demands—and that's probably why we're seeing more of these relationships.

We're very youth-oriented in this country, and I'm not sure it's a compliment, but in order to stay pretty, it sometimes helps to clean up a little area that can't be helped through diet and exercise, so I believe in plastic surgery. Anything that man has learned to make us look better longer is good. I think it has to be done gently though; you don't want to look like someone else. However, for me, I think plastic surgery is just about taboo because I'm afraid of keloids, so I'll have to rely on care as long as possible.

My skin seems to be getting better with time, and I think it's because of my diet, exercise, and the vitamins I take—a daily multivitamin preparation plus vitamins C and A, which I increase in bad weather. I also take garlic tablets that are made in Japan, and they have made a difference in my skin. Cleansing is very important, and if my skin is dry, I increase my vitamin A and it helps. These days I use makeup to embellish rather than to conceal, because by accenting instead of trying to cover up distinctive, though possibly irregular, features, a woman can attain truly striking individuality.

When thinking about food, you have to get rid of the word "diet"—the way you eat is either a life-style or it isn't. "Diet" can be exciting if your goal is more important to you than eating. And you're very lucky if you can maintain the discipline to watch what you eat, because it's rather boring. I don't eat a big breakfast because I find that I can go longer during the day when I don't eat and then enjoy a lovely early dinner. I know breakfast is essential, but I only have a little piece of bran toast, freshly squeezed grapefruit juice, and Sanka, or when I'm under a lot of pressure, camomile tea. I like an early dinner because I find it gives my body a longer time to digest food and I rest better at night. Most of what I eat is now broiled—although I used to think that broiled meant boring. I also give in to my body when it makes certain demands—like one for meat. When I want steak, I have it. But usually I only eat meat six to eight times a year, and then calf's liver or, once in a while, veal. I love wine and drink it every night, even when I'm dining alone. It complements my food and I'm quite serious about it.

Although I don't have a formal exercise routine, I feel that exercise is necessary and can notice the difference when I don't get any. I work out the lazy man's way—when I wake up in the morning, I put a towel on the floor and do sit-ups for seven minutes. I do the same at night. I'm very lucky to be in good shape, but part of the reason is the work I do, which is very hard. I wear very high heels and they are wonderful for the legs. I have to breathe very deeply and that's wonderful for the chest.

Women can improve with age if they nurture and take care of their minds as well as their bodies and faces. With time, the personality softens. You become more humane and compromise does not become such an unattractive word—it can actually benefit relationships. I was on a rampage when I was younger. I believed in being direct and honest about everything, but I've relaxed a bit from that. I understand human frailty; it applies to me, it applies to everyone. I've learned to laugh a great deal, to take things less seriously than I did at twenty-five, and most important of all, when to remain silent. I feel that I've made peace with that inner struggle and it shows, both mentally and physically.

Part I

Your Attitude After 40

Chapter 1

Philosophy: How Women See Themselves

"I've never had a better time, I've never enjoyed life more, never felt more complete than I do now," declares actress Joan Fontaine. "I think passage on earth is for some sort of self-completion—growth and knowledge and all that. When I was twenty-six, Virgil Thomson told me what a beautiful woman I would someday be. And that philosophy, since I was born in the Orient, is the kind I understand. Youth has a marvelous, fresh, early dawn look about it, but there is tremendous beauty in the late afternoon too." Mary Tyler Moore states, "I have so much more in my heart and my head than I had when I was thirty." Says Elizabeth Ashley, "I think being forty is the best of both worlds: I've had time to gain lots of experience and I still have time to use it well"; and Sophia Loren comments, "If you're happy in life, you should not be afraid or ashamed of your wrinkles."

All over forty, all better than ever in a variety of ways, these well-known women prove that beauty has less to do with age than it does with the kind of attitude that allows them to take life and change in stride.

The way you feel about yourself shapes everything you do, including the way you look. We all know women who act as if they are attractive, and whether or not they are, because they think they are we find them attractive as well. Owing to the enormous shift in the age of the population now, which is slowly but surely making its impact felt in all areas, beauty standards are in a state of flux. But one fact remains constant—that beauty is an attitude, an overall impression that includes every part of you, your looks and health as well as your mind. Statistically, the median age of women is rising. Women forty and over, once the neglected segment of the public, are soon to be center stage, the majority. Now they can change their image, which has been, for the most part, a negative one.

It's sometimes difficult to feel positive about change when the grown-up woman is not a power symbol in our culture. Although the middle years can be a glorious time for many women—those who do not measure themselves by society's yardstick—for many others who have learned the stereotype, they are just the opposite. Explains Dr. Jan Sinnott, a psychologist at the Gerontology Research Center of the National Institute on Aging and an associate professor at Towson State University, "A woman has to be aware that her roles will change. She might notice that society often doesn't think highly of a mature woman. She might not be valued much by some men as a sex object after forty. Being a wife and mother might be less important since children are leaving home. As a worker, she might be caught in a low-paying, nonexecutive job. And lots of women will not be able to change this basic situation. One thing they shouldn't be doing is blaming themselves, though. . . . These are attitude problems on the part of society. Wanting to look eighteen when one is forty-five, for example," she comments, "is a silly and unrealistic goal even though a sexist society fosters it . . . being forty-five is not a woman's 'fault,' but an accomplishment. It's far more positive for women to develop and live up to their private goals as women than to engage in the futile struggle to live up to the goals assigned to them by this society." She continues that instead of talking about role losses, women can look at new role choices they are free to accept after forty. And instead of internalizing society's standards, they can choose their own standards. Says she, "The distinctive, individual, mature face is beautiful—maybe more so than the fresh but look-alike one—and the experienced personality has more to offer than the childlike one. Society—not the mature woman—has to be redone."

THE MEANINGLESSNESS OF FORTY

It's important to realize that forty is a number of our own creation, an imposed cutoff—for being young, for being beautiful, since our culture usually equates beauty with youth. Biologically, the number forty is not meaningful. Physiological changes at this age are continuations of those that started some twenty years earlier, as you'll learn in Chapter 3, and menopause for most does not occur for another ten years. Society has traditionally valued women for their ability to bear and rear children—not for their skill and professional worth—and by forty they are presumably finished with childbearing, so their worth has diminished. If we look back in American history, this is certainly the case. In their book *We, the American Women*, authors Beth Millstein and Jeanne Bodin point out that in the 1700s old maids were maligned, portrayed as "peevish, conceited, disagreeable, hypocritical . . . never to be pleased, good for nothing creatures." Old World attitudes about a woman's position in society remained the same in the New World: even though law allowed single women and widows greater freedom and legal rights than married women, they often chose to marry because European religious and social tradition dictated that marriage was the only natural state; women could only find happiness and meaning in life as wives and mothers. Also, there were not many opportunities for women to support themselves, so rather than becoming financial burdens on male relatives, they married. Later, in frontier society, large families were needed to get all the work done, so women were expected to bear as many children as possible—the average family included at least seven. This frequent childbearing, however, considering the conditions of life, was dangerous to women's health, so many died young. Ironically, "The belief that women were healthiest when they were housewives and mothers remained strong throughout the decade of the 1950's, in spite of the conflicting realities," state Millstein and Bodin. "When she was 32, the average woman's last child was in school. With a life expectancy of 77 years, she had 45 'leftover' years to live." The "leftover" years—a phrase we still live with—is more invalid than ever, now that so many women are proving that there is not only life after forty but love, beauty, excitement, challenge, achievement, and so much more.

Comparing then and now, Virginia Sadock, M.D., an associate professor of psychiatry at the New York University Medical Center, claims, "Thirty or forty years ago, women were very secure in their positions at age forty. They might have had a harder time in terms of feeling the loss of youth and attractiveness than women of forty do today, because plastic surgery was not as acceptable and physical fitness was not emphasized, so that in certain narcissistic ways it may have been harder. But the divorce rate was much lower, and even if you weren't happily married, you were secure in your position as a wife and you felt respected as such." She explains that this subservient position led to other difficulties—those of seeing children leave home while you were still quite young because you started so much younger to have

them than women do today. "And in that respect, I think it is easier for women now," Dr. Sadock observes. "Women are having children later or not having children. One thing they deal with that men do not is coming to the end of their procreative function." And while menopause is usually much after forty, she points out, women don't think of having children at forty-seven or forty-eight. "Career, work, is a tremendous factor in terms of helping women through change. You feel yourself to be a productive, valuable member of society in terms of the work that you do, and that was not so thirty or forty years ago."

Dr. Sadock points to economic independence as a major factor in making forty more acceptable. "Some of the things that enable older men to be socially accepted—power, experience, and position, rather than the magnetism of their youth—are privileges extended to women now," she asserts. "The age at which women can have children has been medically extended. Women take good care of themselves . . . they are not physically worn out by age forty. Women have more resources at hand with which to cope with the process of aging."

MIDLIFE CRISIS

"I had been warned that there was some major rite of passage involved in turning forty," says Susan Strasberg. "But I was so busy writing that I didn't even notice it. There's supposedly a standard way to feel at every age and I think that's nonsense." What then of midlife crisis?

Don't all women experience one? It seems that they don't—or at least not necessarily at forty. Some experience it at thirty, or forty, or in relation to things that have nothing to do with age, and any major change might trigger it—"children leaving home, the job market, when they decide to change careers, it varies," says Dr. Sadock. Brooke Hayward admits, "It was far more difficult approaching forty than actually reaching it. I really had to reevaluate my entire life in a way that perhaps, with youth and carelessness, one simply doesn't do." Adds Dr. Sadock, "In a very healthy way, this midlife crisis is simply a reevaluation of what you have done, a stocktaking that you should do every so often regardless of age. In a more distressing way, it manifests itself in depression, extreme anxiety, panic, and regression." Elsa Peretti, the jewelry designer, went through the latter and tells how turning forty was a trauma for her: "It is maturity. You find you have less time to do the things you want and whatever looks you had are starting to fade . . . you accept it only if you are satisfied with your life, as I now think I am."

Perhaps, then, the most positive step you can take is to transform the concept of midlife crisis to midlife checkpoint, and use forty, as it has been used throughout time, throughout history, as a marker, as exactly that. No more, no less. After forty you still have half of your life left, explains Dr. Sinnott, who adds that women as a group are survivors with a long life-span, so it's essential to look at your goals and reevaluate them if they are not working:

but they have to be realistic. For example, while you can minimize changes in shape, there will be some changes that will occur anyway because you are metabolizing differently. She stresses that change is a part of life and there's nothing wrong or bad about it except if we decide that we want to be exactly as we were before.

To underscore this further Dr. Sadock states that a woman can stay her best by not investing everything in outward appearances. The analogy she suggests is that of a lovely piece of furniture. You can worry that someone will put a cigarette burn on it, you can be concerned about every crack, or you can enjoy the history that goes along with living with it by saying that this particular mark came from a fabulous party, that burn from the cigarette of a dear old friend. "It's a variation on beauty is in the eye of the beholder," she says. "If you define beauty as always being fresh and young, there's no way that anyone can stay that way when she gets old. By the same token, if you think of beauty as character, expression, warmth of feeling and experience, then you're of value."

Helen Gurley Brown, who has devoted her life to shaping attitudes through the pages of *Cosmopolitan* magazine, figures it this way: "Women 'disapprove' with age in many areas—you will never be as firm and scrumptious and creamy again as you were at twenty or even thirty. This *hurts*. It is absurd to say you don't miss the succulent, not-too-far-from-perfection you had *then*. Nevertheless, you just *about* compensate and sometimes more than compensate with your brain and your poise and your actual *enjoyment* of life. People love to be with you now, you are not half dead over some dopey man who didn't deserve such adoration; the man you *do* love and go to bed with can be absolutely marvelous; if you have achieved in your career, all the rewards start flowing in and they are *considerable* . . . money, success, recognition and happiness every day over that particular work.''

It's interesting that when you ask a woman over forty if she wants to return to twenty again, you may get a surprising response. If her life has not been terrible, most times she'll refuse, saying twenty was too hard. Or she'll qualify her answer, saying yes, but only if she could know what she knows now. ''I wasn't happy at twenty,'' says Joan Fontaine. ''I was miserable. I wouldn't mind physically being twenty, but not mentally or emotionally. It's such a pity that youth is given to the young. It would be lovely now, when the body is not as elastic.'' Explains Audrey Hepburn, ''When I think of myself at twenty—I was very much at sea; not at all sure what life was all about. With time, you gain a certain degree of maturity; you've made choices; you've done so much.''

AGING WITHOUT GROWING OLD

If you look at those vital women who age without growing old, you'll notice that they all have traits in common. They are *curious*, they seek ever-expanding frontiers, new challenges. Declares Jill St. John, ''Now I realize that attaining your goals isn't as important as striving for them.'' They are *involved:* with work, paid or volunteer, with studies or hobbies. Says Joan Fontaine, ''I'm doing one thousand things . . . lecturing on Chinese art, pursuing many other interests, including television and stage projects. That's what keeps someone young!'' Plus— and very important—they *keep fit and active* because flexibility applies to the muscles as well as the mind. It's actually moot as to whether your attitude shapes your looks or your looks shape your attitude, because success breeds success. Take off those ten pounds, exercise away those ten inches, care for your skin the way it needs caring for, correct your hair color, and you'll view the world differently—because everyone will view you in a new way. And while it does not necessarily hurt to be beautiful, after forty, for most, it's no accident. Jane Fonda has a body as lithe as a teen-ager's, but she stays in enviable shape by exercising constantly. Dancer Juliet Prowse, while acknowledging that she's not capable of some of the moves she made at twenty, notices that her stamina is much better now because she's stayed in shape for so many years. ''Every day I take two hours of ballet class, swim, take my three dogs for two very long walks, and do yoga. And of course, I still dance professionally.'' Angie Dickinson confesses, ''Health is my top priority. I'm a big believer in nutrition and study it continually. I avoid food with additives, preservatives, and food coloring. I also work out for ten to fifteen minutes each day on a treadmill." Model Carmen swims, Sunny Griffin dances for two hours a day, and Polly Bergen bicycles and does calisthenics. Ali MacGraw keeps her fabulous looks and slim body by eating lightly, exercising often, trying to relax, and following an in-depth moisturizing skin-care program for her dry complexion. "My skin is really in good condition and I think that completely relates to the care I've always taken with it."

FEELING GOOD ABOUT YOURSELF

"The gift of youth is that you don't worry about aging," explains Dr. Sadock. "You have that sense of omnipotence that you don't have when you reach forty because you've seen the time go by. Thinking that you can live forever, do anything, that all options are open to you, that you'll always be healthy, is no longer true, because you've gained experience. You face decreasing abilities, and that's what creates some of the difficulties of aging." She stresses that the important thing is to feel good emotionally, to take care of yourself in a healthy way, to participate in some physical activity and if you can, to do a lot of things that you like to do. A suggestion she offers for further boosting your self-esteem is to make lists to remind yourself of your value and of all the productive and positive things you've done.

The experts agree that you have to come to grips with reorganizing your goals—you may have achieved so much, but your limits are no longer the same. Ask yourself where your limits are. Then try to achieve these and to enjoy them—to take pleasure in yourself. "You may feel like your stomach is no longer as flat as it once was," says Dr. Sadock, "but if you ask yourself what made it change, hopefully it was not just gluttony, but something that made you feel good; perhaps taking care of other people so that you just didn't have time to invest in yourself; or having children, if it was a worthwhile experience for you. If you have lines around your eyes, hopefully they came from smiling, or frowning, or experiencing life. They are signs that you've lived. You can stay content with your age by feeling a certain way about yourself. And it also helps if you are appreciated; and if you can't get appreciation from a mate, go out and seek it from friends and accomplishments."

Chapter 2

Psychology: How Men See Women

"I've always said that what makes a woman most attractive is thinking she is," says Burt Reynolds. "It may sound corny, but the essence of beauty to me, both physical and spiritual, really does come from within." Among his "ideal" women are actresses Jane Fonda and Carol Burnett. "There's no question that the woman of forty or forty plus is a woman of great allure—she's developed her own personal style and assurance—and really *cares* how she looks. I feel that she has a sense of adventure about herself," adds designer Bill Blass. Actor Robert Stack claims that Lauren Bacall exemplifies the type of women he finds most appealing—a woman who likes herself and has a "feminine presence without being arrogant; strength without militance." Explains photographer Francesco Scavullo, "A young girl . . . only has to wear a smile and a pair of jeans to look smashing. But I really admire older women who continue to look healthy, sexy, vital. . . ." He lists Jacqueline Onassis, Lee Radziwill, and Maxine de la Falaise as prime examples.

It's evident that just as women after forty are changing, so are the ways in which men see them. There will probably be more change on the way as women become less con-

strained by both age and image and more self-assured and confident. Contrast a forty-five-year-old of today who really takes care of herself, and believes she can look better than she ever did, with one of just ten years ago and the difference might amaze you. Today she has more options in every area, and most important, she's taking advantage of them. "There's a totally different attitude now. Women have learned the necessity and desirability of physical fitness. Their thinking about children and their relevance to the success of marriage has changed," opines Harold Glasser, president of Miss Universe, Inc., and executive producer of the Miss Universe and Miss America pageants. To explain the present he refers to the past, when a woman married at an early age with the immediate objective of raising a family and concentrated entirely on the home. Then, says he, it was the rare woman who could maintain her figure, who had the opportunity to follow world events and voice opinions about them. After dinner, women would go into another room for "woman talk," while men would congregate in the parlor with brandy and cigars to discuss current situations. Today, however, women don't retire to a different room, he

/13

continues. They are involved, aware, well-educated. And these are the reasons that he, although often surrounded by the world's most gorgeous, most nubile young girls, prefers older women. "Since a person is the sum total of every experience, the most interesting people are those who have the opportunity to develop," he states. "A woman who has reached the age of forty has . . . she's built a career, sharpened viewpoints, traveled and had relationships, so for me, she's a very interesting person."

THE AGE OF BEAUTY

From his vantage point of observing beauty through the years, Glasser maintains that it is no longer the sine qua non that it might have been in the past, when artifice was looked upon unfavorably, so a woman could not make the most of her looks. "Today, we accept almost everything," he says, stressing that what a woman makes of herself is more important than physical beauty with nothing behind it. Designer Giorgio Sant' Angelo says, "Women can get more beautiful with age—and handsome women get fabulous; strong features last a long time." He emphasizes that looks have a direct relationship with attitude, understanding; everything comes from the mind, the character. "The women I know who are 'beautiful' after forty have sex appeal . . . vitality, like . . . Lena Horne." Growing older but not aging is, to him, taking care of yourself men-

tally and emotionally. Keeping up with life and never thinking of retiring or taking up needlepoint at home.

"I think that a certain amount of narcissism is healthy," says psychiatrist Virginia Sadock. "But our culture does outrageous things to women. The idea of not being able to have a wrinkle or gray in your hair is ridiculous. It's perpetuated by the advertising industry and I think it really has to be counteracted by women." Counteraction starts by being truthful about your age, says she, so that people see that over forty does not necessarily look "old." She uses as an example feminist Germaine Greer, who at forty-six was told during a television interview that she did not look her age, and replied that this was the way forty-six-year-old women look now. "Women who lie do themselves a great disservice," continues Dr. Sadock. "Because once they start telling the truth, they indeed have aged a great deal."

THE NEED TO PLEASE

"The biggest problem a woman has with her hair now is her husband—how he feels about it, about her," observes hair stylist Michael Mazzei. Women want the approval of men. In our culture this attitude is traditional, involved in large part with social and economic dependency. Women are often considered adornments, possessions, symbols of a man's status in life. While it seems like a perfectly normal course of action for a woman to make herself attractive for a man, it's often complicated by her motivation for doing so. If she feels she *has* to—when choice is removed—the action can be considered manipulative or exploitive. This exploitive element between men and women is evident in many aspects of life; a hairstyle is one, weight is another. Kim Chernin, author of *The Obsession: Reflections on the Tyranny of Slenderness,* claims that our male-dominated culture calls for women to be slender to unconsciously limit the symbolic physical expression of her power. She explains that in America the physical ideal for a woman is a man's body, so it is no wonder that women are the truly obsessive dieters: they are trying to diet away their curves and roundness because shape involves issues of identity and place in society. Voluptuousness is acceptable only when women are not trying to change their social status. When they claim power and independence, men respond differently and culture demands a return to a boyish silhouette. In summary, she believes that by making themselves appear less female, women are symbolically asking for the social rights reserved traditionally for men. The fact that society wants a mature woman to look like an adolescent girl indicates cultural anxiety about female power.

As women are moving away from those roles that traditionally gave them status, they may still seek approval—but out of choice this time and due to a new independence built in part by economic self-sufficiency. "It makes much less difference to me now if my husband gives me the go-ahead," states one forty-three-year-old, who has been working for the last five years. "I'm not going to fall apart if he doesn't like what I do." Says Estelle Fuchs in *The Second Season,* "Today's woman is in a sense a pioneer, for never before have so many been faced with the prospect of living out their lives without the traditional roles that charted the course of their aging." She goes on to say that women are not going to go back to traditional systems, although the independence of being single, childless, and having physical autonomy might not be as ideal as they had imagined. But, by the same token, they are not about to fall apart at the prospect of creating new roles and life-styles.

We're in a developing society, an evolving culture, one that in the last ten years has advanced Gloria Steinems and Betty Friedans, as well as a host of others dedicated to improving the lot of all women on all the issues where they've been patronized, ignored, or relegated to a lesser position. And as women achieve a certain status and prove that the years after forty can be a time of beauty and productivity, the families they raise will be free of the attitudes that men, thus society, now have.

OLDER WOMEN, YOUNGER MEN

In a culture that accepts the pairing

of older men with younger women but looks askance at an older woman with a younger man, the increasing frequency of the latter combination is an indication of social change. More women and men both appear to view it as a matter of course. While a difference in age of five or six years is not perceived by many as a difference at all, one of fifteen or twenty years is. However, today biological age and chronological age seem years apart because of the ways women are caring for themselves. "It's not the quality of the skin that counts for me, it's the quality of the woman," explains a man in his late twenties regarding his relationship with a forty-two-year-old woman. "She is stimulating and sure of herself. She offers me a richness by virtue of her experience."

Certainly a man's image of a woman's desirability is very individual, conditioned by what he is accustomed to. We're creatures of our environment, thus we tend to continue those attitudes that influenced us as children. Comments Giorgio Sant' Angelo, "I've always felt that a younger man and an older woman had a much better relationship. I've seen it work in my own family and it has a lot to do with the intelligence of the woman." And a physical relationship to him is very important. "It's unfortunate that society feels a woman is finished when she can't have children anymore,"

he says disapprovingly. "The secret of life is keeping up . . . in all areas. And that includes a sex life as well."

FORTY AND ITS ADVANTAGES

Ask a man to sum up why he finds you so special now, and he might answer with a comparison as Harold Glasser does, that the advantage of being twenty-five is obviously youth—and all that youth means: the carefree attitude about health, about age, about your figure that you take for granted since you don't see the changes that age can bring. But after forty a woman is free from the concerns and anxieties and the feelings of inadequacy that a twenty-five-year-old has. "I think this woman has achieved the confidence of development, of success in a career, of encounters with men and the problems they have presented," Glasser responds. "She's survived some of her choices and will go on to make others." This only proves what many of us already know: that we have strengths and desirable qualities at every stage in life—youth, middle age, and old age. It's a matter of making the most of them. After forty, experience and everything positive that accompanies it are your assets—and the future can be even better!

Chapter 3

Physiology

"Aging is not a sudden process that starts at forty. It begins practically when adolescence ends, and it's so gradual and natural throughout life that we are almost unaware of it," explains psychologist Jan Sinnott. "To me, aging is experiencing the passage of time, but not necessarily deteriorating. Most of the debilitating physical processes that we call aging are really disease processes." She emphasizes that old age starts at seventy-five, when we see dramatic changes in physical characteristics that matter a great deal for most people, and draws attention to the enormous time-span between seventy-five and forty, the age when you start to think about changes that have been happening since you were twenty.

Of course, change on all levels is inevitable—and usually welcome. "Change is part of life," stresses Dr. Sinnott. "You *should* change!" But happily certain changes are avoidable. While we know that no one can stay young forever, we also know that we can delay the aging process through diet, exercise, and the sort of positive attitude that motivates us to stay involved with life, with our looks. We can fine-tune this intimate connection between the mind and the body to our greatest advantage.

INVESTING IN YOURSELF

This is an especially challenging time both physically and mentally, as more doors are opening for women careerwise and otherwise, and with them more options for staying fit and conditioned. Today, particularly, beauty is synonymous with health, vitality, dynamism, qualities that can only be achieved by stimulating your mind *and* body, by investing in yourself. By investing in your mind, you'll improve your psychological and intellectual abilities—which can expand at every age—and by investing in your body, you'll offset a decline in your physical abilities that will happen if no action is taken.

The first step, agree the experts, is to *start moving*. Use your body or lose it. Stressful exercise is particularly important after forty, not only to keep your shape but to prevent osteoporosis (bone loss) and raise declining estrogen levels. Dr. Sarah Roshan, a clinical instructor in obstetrics and gynecology at Albert Einstein College of Medicine and in private practice in Millburn, New

Jersey, explains that these changes, which started at age twenty, resulting in a decrease in the heart's output, blood flow through the kidneys, and oxygen consumption, can be counteracted—if we train our bodies with the right breathing and strenuous exercise. In addition, staying taut and firm through exercise puts you in control—a wonderful plus for your state of mind.

Next step, *stop eating.* You need less food through the years, but whatever you eat has to do more nutritionally. To provide the energy and sense of well-being you seek, look toward the freshest of fruits and vegetables, fish and chicken instead of red meat, sufficient calcium—found in low-fat milk and cheese—and plenty of fluids to replace a decreasing water content in the body, especially in the cells, that accompanies aging. In the pure cosmetic sense, remember too that eating the wrong foods can result in depression, fatigue, and irritability, all of which show up on your face!

PREGNANCY NOW

Believing that she could be a wiser, better mother now because she feels more secure about herself, more in touch, is the way one woman sums up childbearing at age forty-three. Whether it's because they've married later, been absorbed by a career, or simply felt they were not ready for a child before, women are having children after forty—and the option is still open. In fact, it's estimated that 95 percent of women at this age can ex-pect to have healthy offspring without any major problem. However, changes brought about by age can result in problems and should be considered.

According to Dr. Roshan, chromosomal abnormality increases with age, so an amniocentesis is necessary. This test, administered during pregnancy, allows your physician to detect, thus act against, potential complications. It involves the removal of a sample of amniotic fluid through the abdomen to read the chromosomal makeup of the baby. "Because the rate of fertility goes down after thirty-five, it's harder to conceive," she continues. "The ovaries have started to age and the amount of estrogen/progesterone they produce is less than when you were in your twenties." The incidence of miscarriage and of delivery by caesarian section is higher after forty, as are the possibilities of an elevation in blood pressure, edema, and proteinuria (protein in the urine) occurring late in pregnancy, usually during the eighth or ninth month. These complications can happen earlier depending on a woman's condition, says Dr. Roshan, who emphasizes that termination of pregnancy is the only "treatment" for this condition, known as preeclampsia. She's observed as well that pregnant women over forty require more rest in general and more strenuous dieting and exercise to get their bodies back in shape after childbirth. These days the optimum weight-gain during pregnancy is considered to be between twenty and twenty-eight pounds, and since good nutrition is vital for the baby's development, a diet sufficient in protein, vegetables, and fresh fruit is strongly recommended.

MENOPAUSE—THE PHYSIOLOGICAL ASPECT

One of the major changes in a woman's life between the ages of forty-five and fifty-five—the exact year depends upon the individual heredity pattern and gynecological history—is menopause. And like all rites of passage it has a psychological aspect as well as a physiological one: the acceptance of the family, of society at large, can complicate this transition or smooth it. But studies indicate that of the twenty or thirty possible physical complaints associated with hormonal changes during menopause, there are only two reliable changes that occur in the majority of women—hot flushes and cessation of menstruation. All of the rest happen to only a fraction of women.

Despite this truth—that menopause for the majority poses no physical problem—many, including women themselves, are quick to dismiss any health complaint as associated with climacteric (the whole group of changes that appear at midlife). Dr. Sinnott observes, "It's a sad story that many true physical problems that women bring to their doctors are simply diagnosed as symptoms of menopause and ignored . . . or treated with tranquilizers." Although some women stop menstruating abruptly, others experience a more gradual shift, irregularities in their cycle that may continue for many years. These can make them nervous or anxious and with good cause. As anthropologist Estelle Fuchs explains in *The Second Season,* a period of unexpected and irregular bleeding after some thirty-odd years of fairly regular and familiar menstruation can justifiably cause worry and panic. Many women fear that irregular bleeding can be an early symptom of uterine cancer, or of polyps or other growths. A missed period could signal pregnancy—since it's possible to still conceive up to about a year after one's last period. Happily, most women take menopause in stride. Generally those who are happy with themselves, who are achievers and successful in life, do not have complaints, observes Dr. Sarah Roshan. "But when there are symptoms of change of life—which occur in a certain percentage of women—they can be relieved by good nutrition, proper exercise, and psychological support from the woman's physician and family. . . . An actual hormonal deficiency is responsible for only 20 percent of the complaints that women have at this stage of life."

Dr. Roshan explains that problems can arise if the family does not give a woman the acceptance and understanding she needs now, especially since this can be a time of fear of aging, of the unknown, of the inevitability of death. Also responsible for some symptoms are the empty-nest syndrome as well as the fear many women have of losing their husband to a younger woman. "Women should have themselves prepared physically, psychologically, and financially to go through this time with better defenses," she emphasizes, which is why she advises the young to prepare for forty when they are twenty.

ESTROGEN REPLACEMENT THERAPY

A controversial way to treat dramatic climacteric problems, Estrogen Replacement Therapy (ERT) involves taking oral supplements of estrogen to replenish naturally dwindling supplies. Dr. Roshan states, "Osteoporosis can be helped by estrogen to a limited extent, but because it is a growth hormone and can increase the chance of uterine cancer, it should be given by a qualified gynecologist only after a careful evaluation and under close follow-up."

She recommends ERT only if a nonhormonal approach is not effective but prefers to begin with the following nutritional program, which consists of:

• Vitamins: she advises 100 mg. of vitamin B to help women cope better with the stress of everyday life, then 500 mg. of vitamin C plus zinc, which is believed to help keep connective tissues elastic and build the system's defense against virus and infection. She prescribes 50 micrograms of selenium to help vitamin absorption, plus 200 to 400 IUs of vitamin E, a natural preservative that is thought to keep blood vessels working well and to relieve vaginal dryness and loss of elasticity.

• Vigorous exercise: she explains that exercise releases the estrogen naturally stored in body fat, changing it into a form the body can use, and also builds up bones.
• Diet: she counsels a diet rich in calcium to overcome bone loss after forty (if calcium intake is low, supplements are advised), as well as plenty of fresh fruits and vegetables, three to five eggs per week if cholesterol is not high, and limited amounts of red meat.

If the preceding approach does not produce the desired results, she may prescribe the nonhormonal drug *Bellergal S*—a combination of the sedative phenobarbital and antihistamines—to treat hot flushes, headaches, tension, and other complaints. To combat vaginal dryness she begins with a water-soluble preparation and if it's not effective, continues with an estrogen cream.

As a last resort Dr. Roshan suggests a short-term estrogen program, tailored for the individual and constantly monitored—only if there is no history of cancer in the family, and in the lowest possible dosage that will relieve the symptoms. The monitoring includes careful checkups: every six months a Pap smear and a thermogram for breast screening; every year an endometrial biopsy to check endometrial tissue. She emphasizes that monitored long-term hormone therapy can be harmful, since estrogen treatment increases the incidence of hypertension five to eight times and the possibility of breast and uterine cancer three- to five-fold. Of course, being or having been treated with estrogen does not necessarily mean that you will get cancer. It does mean, however, that you and your physician must decide carefully whether the benefits of ERT outweigh its risks.

There is a question in some minds about the extent of the benefits of ERT. Influenced by recent studies, Dr. Jan Sinnott feels that many of the useful effects of ERT are not that dramatic. She mentions that while it reduces hot flushes, many women report that when they have stopped therapy, their flushes have returned twice as strong; in the case of osteoporosis only some women are helped, and to a limited extent. And vaginal dryness, often eased by estrogen, can be treated satisfactorily with nonhormonal lubricants.

MENOPAUSE—THE ATTITUDINAL ASPECT

While menopause in the past might have been considered the major event in a woman's life after forty, studies indicate that at present this view is no longer prevalent. In fact, one of the greatest negatives associated with menopause—that a woman could no longer have children—is currently perceived by many as a positive feature. Many women have had all the children they wanted and are tired of bothering with menstruation and birth control or worrying about pregnancy. In the past menopause was certainly more traumatic when children left home and a woman lost her major role as mother. But the motherhood aspect is less pronounced for

many of today's women who have developed other interests in life and want this time to pursue them actively. Many women who are mothers had their children at an earlier age so they in turn are younger when their role shifts—in their thirties rather than their forties and fifties—so that they've had a number of years to make an adjustment and to assume other roles. Many of these women report that their marriages are actually better now that they have time alone with their mates—thus menopause is often cited as a source of sexual renewal.

SEX CAN BE BETTER THAN EVER

It's a fact that a woman's sex drive does not diminish as she ages; she can remain sexually active throughout her life. And for many women, sexual pleasure actually increases with age. The reason for this is largely emotional, say the experts, who point to a woman's confidence, experience, and familiarity with her body—its needs and responses. By her forties too she's shed old guilts and anxieties about sex, so that she's more comfortable with her sexuality. She may, as well, simply have more time to devote to her mate, to herself. "I've been able to involve myself more with my husband these days—to get to know him again—and this has made us more intimate sexually," explains one woman in her fifties. "I'm exercising now and doing more of the things I like. My husband seems more interested in me as a result—and our sex life has been more emotionally rewarding," observes another.

Intensified feelings of self-worth and competence that are associated with a job that's going well or other satisfactory accomplishments can also boost sexual enthusiasm and interest. And the physical complaints that occur with menopause—vaginal dryness and painful intercourse—can be easily alleviated by treatment with a lubricant so that they are not deterrents.

Part of this sexual vitality after forty is attributed to physiology, the theory being that the more the body gets used to arousal and orgasm, the easier it is to get a response. Again, too, attitude is cited—if a woman has led a happy life, is satisfied with herself, she'll enjoy sex to a greater degree now because she's more confident and less anxious. She knows that she has the capacity to satisfy both her partner and herself.

Famous Faces After 40

There's beauty at every age, as eleven of the world's most recognized and attractive women prove. Here's the way they looked in their twenties and thirties—and now, in their forties, fifties, and sixties.

Raquel Welch

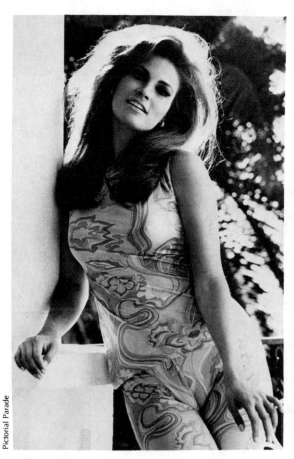

Pictorial Parade

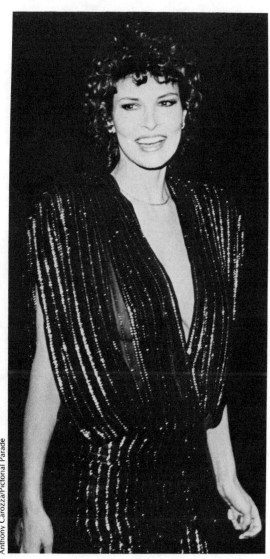

Anthony Carozza/Pictorial Parade

Jacqueline Onassis

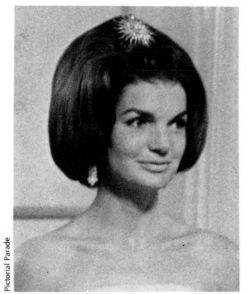

Pictorial Parade

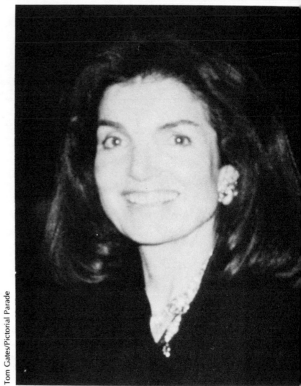

Tom Gates/Pictorial Parade

Brigitte Bardot

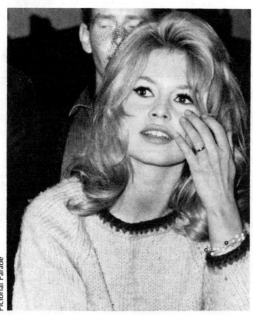

Pictorial Parade

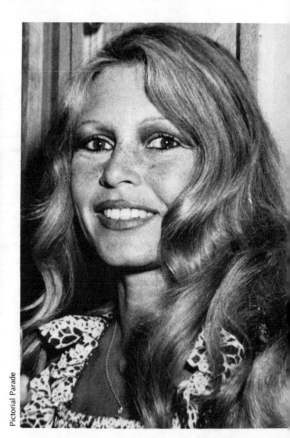

Pictorial Parade

Lauren Bacall

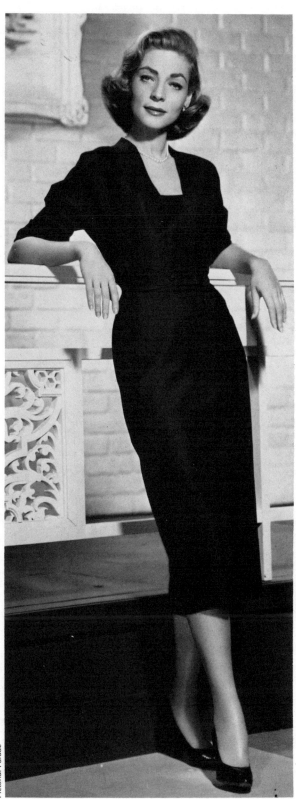

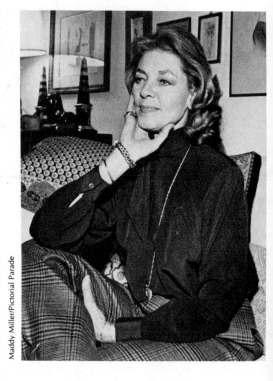

Sophia Loren

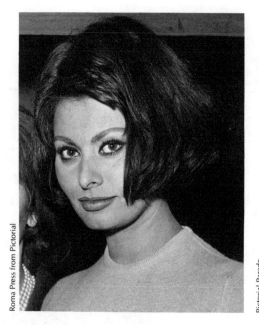

Roma Press from Pictorial

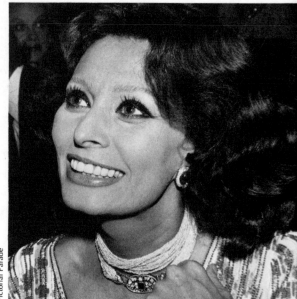

Pictorial Parade

Audrey Hepburn

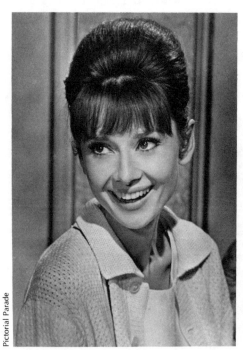

Pictorial Parade

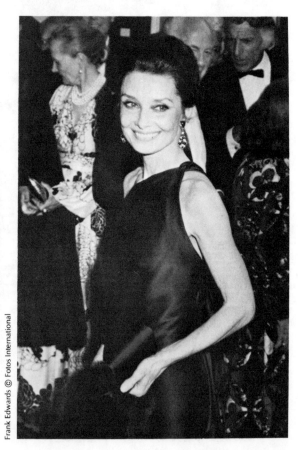

Frank Edwards © Fotos International

Angie Dickinson

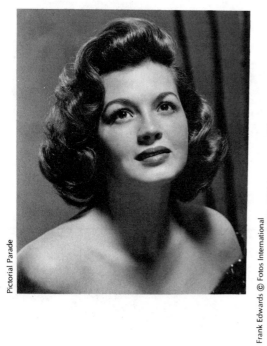

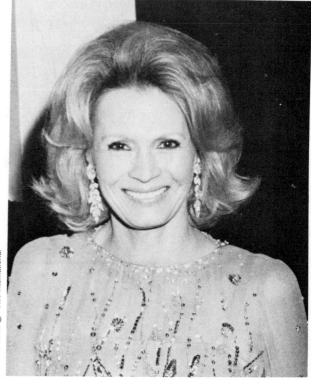

Jane Fonda

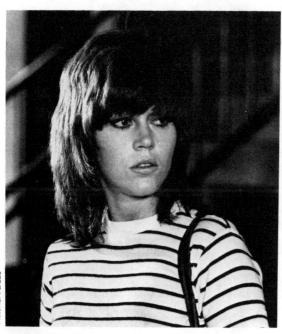

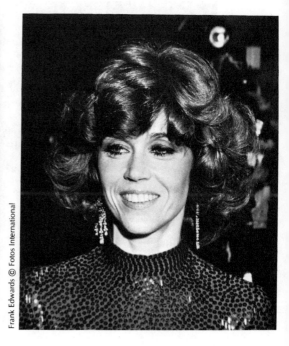

Elizabeth Taylor

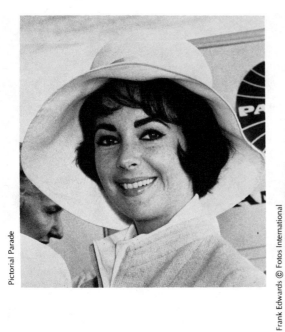

Pictorial Parade

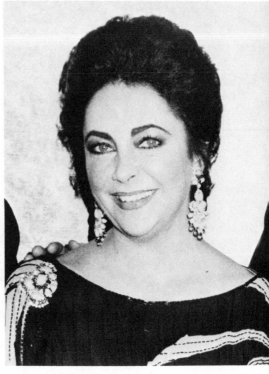

Frank Edwards © Fotos International

Ali MacGraw

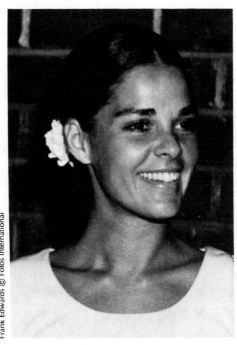

Frank Edwards © Fotos International

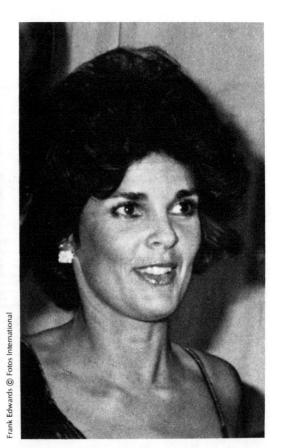

Frank Edwards © Fotos International

Lena Horne

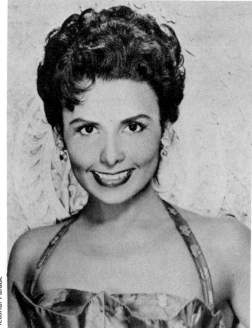

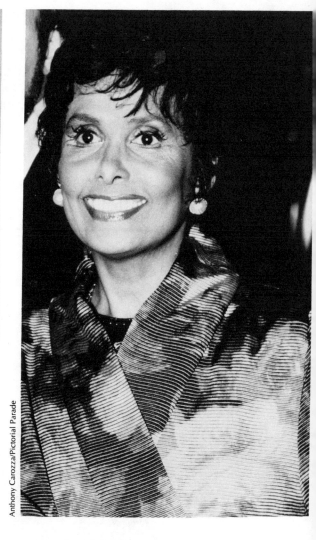

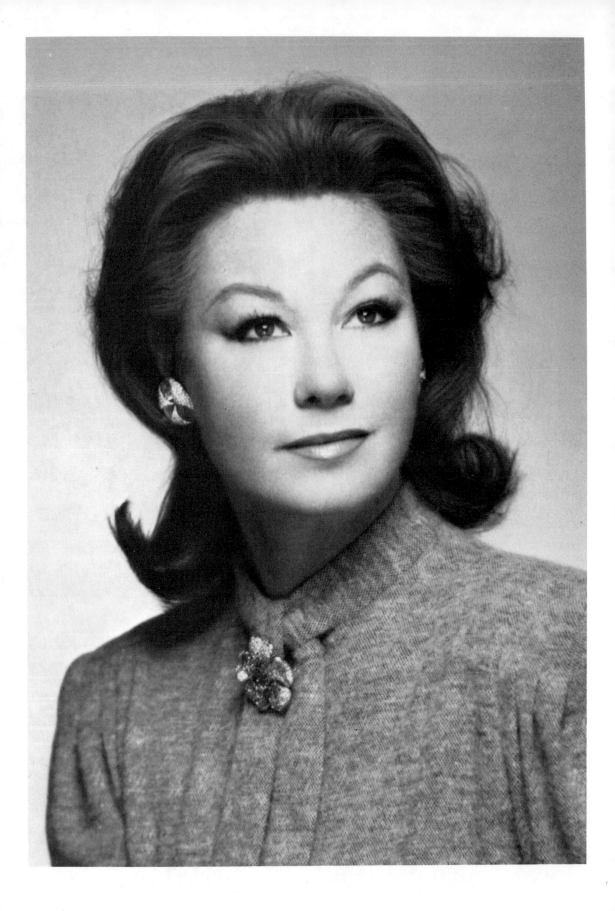

Baroness Nadine de Rothschild

Wife of the Baron Edmond de Rothschild

I think youth is a state of mind—but you have to exercise your mind. For me, the most beautiful time in a woman's "career" is after forty. You become different. If something in your life bothers you, try to change or eliminate it. And if the man you are with is not very attentive anymore, remember there's always someone else. All of the men my husband and I know have started new lives—and all have chosen women over forty!

I was an actress when I met my husband. I think I always had a star guiding me. I never believed in those romantic novels about the typist who married a prince, though—I'm just too realistic for that. I always told myself that nothing was going to fall from the sky, and that it was necessary for me to build my own future. Wealth, fortune, I didn't even have the least idea of what they really encompassed. They were so far from my reality. I couldn't even imagine them. I also never really understood what the name Rothschild carried with it—the dynasty, their importance in finance and industry, in history, too, at a certain era.

Anyhow, one evening I went to a dinner party—I hadn't wanted to go because I intended to go to bed early. I was acting at the Théâtre de Paris. It was my night off and I only wanted to sleep. The friend who invited me insisted I come, so I went. The man sitting next to me had blue eyes, a small mustache; I found him very nice, but nothing more. It was Edmond, my future husband. Before midnight, I announced that I was leaving. He left at the same time and walked me to my car. He opened the door for me and when I was seated, bent over and told me, quickly and abruptly, that he felt that I was the woman of his life. It was as simple as that. And we've been married for nineteen years. I am not a woman's liberationist—I want my husband always to have the feeling that he's keeping me, taking care of me.

But I am very involved in my work. Edmond's concerns—the problems of Israel—have become mine as well. I accompany him there whenever he goes. I also oversee three child-care centers founded by my husband's grandmother. I'm the intermediary between Edmond and the doctors at the Rothschild Foundation, a large hospital. Other commitments are the Braille University of Jerusalem, additional organizations, being a consultant to Porthault (the linens manufacturer), and working with the fragrance company Florasynth on scents for the home. We've already created a fragranced candle and are looking into other possibilities.

As for my beauty regimen, I do not follow an exercise plan, but I do walk a lot—and swim. In fact, I always travel with water goggles. Twice a year I go to a spa in Brittany for water therapy. I stay between ten and fifteen days, following a strict vegetarian diet and swimming daily to get back in shape.

I love to eat—and find it very hard to diet. I prefer to eat more, thus weigh more and be happy, than to deprive myself and feel depressed. I always have breakfast and lunch, and because of our involvements and life-style, large dinners too. I drink a liter of water before breakfast and take magnesium pills every day and have for twenty years. I find them indispensable for my skin, my nerves.

I always cleanse my face very well. I've never gone to bed without removing my makeup first, with a cleansing milk. Then I don't use a cream overnight. In the morning I spray my skin with warm water to hydrate it before applying a moisturizer with a hormone base, powder, and the rest of my makeup. I do my own hair but have regular professional manicures, pedicures, and waxing.

I travel often but try to avoid flying at night because I can't sleep well in planes. If I am going to try to sleep, I get undressed and slip into something comfortable—I find that helps a lot. I also eat very lightly and drink water constantly. The air in planes is so drying.

I think one has to have discipline in life—and organization. When I go to sleep late and have to get up early, I try to schedule in a nap during the day. I also eat less so that I don't weigh down my system. I don't drink much alcohol, but water instead. I never—and I don't think any woman should ever— leave home without being made up and perfumed. Likewise, when I get home, I change and bathe, redo my makeup, and try to look attractive for my husband. I believe a woman can do whatever she wants in the bathroom, but she should always look coiffed and groomed for her husband, for her public.

Part II

Your Face After 40

Chapter 4

Makeup Makes the Glamorous Difference

"A woman can't be glamorous until she's over forty—it's as simple as that," says author and beauty authority Stan Place. "Because glamour comes with creating your own style, and that takes time and experience—advantages which a twenty- or thirty-year-old has to wait a decade or two to get, and which a forty-year-old has—she's learned who she is, where she is, and how to carry it off!"

Bravo! You're forty, or more. You've changed, your skin has changed. Your makeup should change as well. Strive for a look that lets your personality shine through. Think glamour—but not necessarily more makeup. Glamour these days means less. Much less often ends up being more.

Now too you want to spend as much time taking your makeup off as you do putting it on—patting, blending, smudging, so there are no edges, no lines (lines are aging), no matter how much or how little makeup you use. Color counts more than ever, but *when* you wear it counts most. Color should change with the season, with the time of day, with the occasion. A full makeup at 9:00 A.M. can ultimately be as ineffective as a lick of lipstick and a fluff of powder at a formal evening event. That's why building

a beautiful makeup makes so much sense.

BUILDING YOUR MAKEUP

Makeup man Rex, renowned for his skill at creating ageless beauty, believes in building a look with the light: gentler in the morning when the light is soft, intensified in the afternoon when the light is stronger, and completely changed in the evening, when dimmer lights and candlelight wash out reds, so makeup must be brighter, rosier. His secret, which can be yours, too, is to match the mood to the moment—remember, glamour is a state of mind.

THE TOOLS

Achieving ageless beauty depends upon your tools as well as your technique—they have to do the most for you, so they should probably change with the seasons, when skin's needs and fashion colors do. In cold weather your complexion is generally drier. Outdoors, the elements, and indoors, overheating, rob it of precious moisture. Your foundation and/or your moisturizer may have to be more emollient, lipstick creamier; you may turn to gloss for its lubricating action. Colors are usually richer and more full-bodied in fall and winter, while in summer they are lighter, cleaner. In warm weather, especially when the humidity is high, your skin may look its best with a sheerer foundation, perhaps a water-based one, or a bronzing gel—which gives the illusion of a tan—topped by gel rouge, for color without any coverage.

But whatever the reason, or the season, these are the bare necessities that no makeup case should be without:

Foundation

Match it to the skin at your jawline; it should blend in without any line of demarcation. Always test the color in daylight—keeping in mind that makeup looks darker in the bottle and lightens as you spread it. You may need a formulation that is a little richer than the one you used years ago, since your skin may be drier. If it is oily or a combination of dry and oily, try a sheerer or water-based product.
- natural face sponge (sometimes called a silk sponge)—for best application

Concealer

Select a sheer-spreading cream or stick, no more than two shades lighter than your skin.

Pressed powder

In a lightweight, translucent shade.
- long-handled sable brush with fat bristles—for fluffing on a sheer film of powder, plus sweeping off excess

Powder blusher

Easiest to apply, longest lasting. Select clear lively shades that complement your coloring and wardrobe. Best: corals, roses, peaches, honeys. Worst: purples, browns, anything with frost.
- long-handled blusher brush—never use the same brush for powder and blush
- round foam sponge—cut in quarters to form wedges for blending your makeup

Powder eye shadow

Always in a matte formulation—shine is aging, plays up lines and wrinkles. Best: neutral shades like taupe, gray, brown, amber, mauve—your coloring plays a part in your choice—plus a highlighter and several fashion colors. Save the softer, subtler tints for day, go brighter at night.
- long-handled eye-shadow brush or sponge applicator
- slim eyeliner brush—for smudging away lines

Eye pencils

One or two in muted shades—brown, gray, mauve, blue—plus a corrective one in light blue.

Mascara

Black is generally too dark; experiment with shades of gray, navy, burgundy, brown.
- eyelash curler—gives eyes a "lift"
- lash comb—for separating lashes after mascara

Eyebrow pencil

Keep it sharp, color light.
- tweezers—for grooming
- brow brush—for smudging pencil strokes

Lip pencil

In the same color as your lipstick.

Lipstick

In soft pretty shades that work with the rest of your makeup. The brighter your mouth, the more neutral you should color the rest of your face. If you like a mere stain of color, try a tinted lipgloss.
- lip brush—for mistake-proof application

THE TECHNIQUE

Avoid a rude awakening by keeping color to a minimum in the morning, then gently sketching it on in the afternoon. Save surprises for the evening, when the light allows you to compensate with a little skillfully applied artifice.

Facing Morning

- Examine your freshly cleansed face in the morning light; get to know it. Decide where you need correction, where you want emphasis. If you cannot make up in daylight, buy a good mirror with artificial lights around it.
- After moisturizing, harmonize facial proportions with lights and shadows. Cover dark circles, spots, and lines with concealing cream. Blend edges with fingertips or a wedge of sponge (you'll find additional problem-solvers later in this chapter).
- Prime your face and even out skin tone with foundation, spread with a barely damp natural sponge over the face and jawline in a downward direction to flatten facial hairs. A damp sponge will help you avoid streaks and makeup excess, providing a sheer, healthy-looking finish.

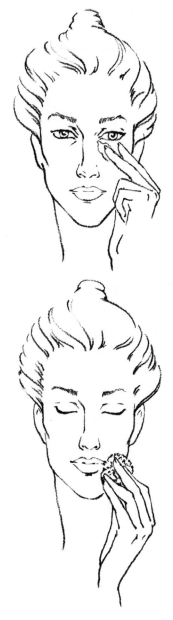

• Dust pressed translucent face powder with a brush lightly over the center of the face and any shiny spots. Brush away excess.

• Blush now, it will make the single biggest change in your look. Smile, then blend color high on the apples of the cheeks with your blusher brush. Bring blusher up along the cheekbone and out to the hairline. Blend all edges with a wedge of sponge. Your goal is a wash of color as if you awakened with it.

• Eyes next; color them neutral in eye-shadow hues of heather, gray, taupe, amber—and lightly over your eyelid only. Whiten them with a line of pale blue pencil along lower inner lash rims; lift them by curling your lashes, then stroking two to three coats of mascara over them; separate the lashes with a lash comb. Feather brows lightly with brow pencil, then brush them straight up and to the sides to smudge the strokes.

• Add glow with lip color—you need it to finish your face—in a soft, clear tint that is in the same color family as your cheeks. Stay away from pearled formulations that play up wrinkles. Red with a touch of blue will make teeth look whiter. Outline lips with pencil, fill in with lipstick, working from the center of the lips out toward each side. Blot lightly and reapply. If you like a sheerer stain of color, try lining lips, smudging the line with your fingertips, then filling in with a tinted lipgloss. Blot.

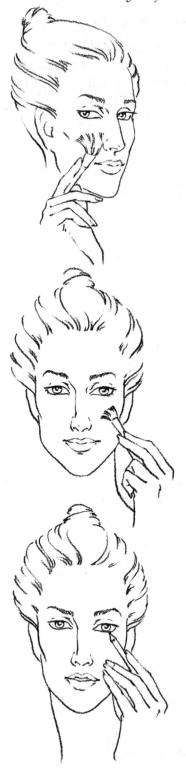

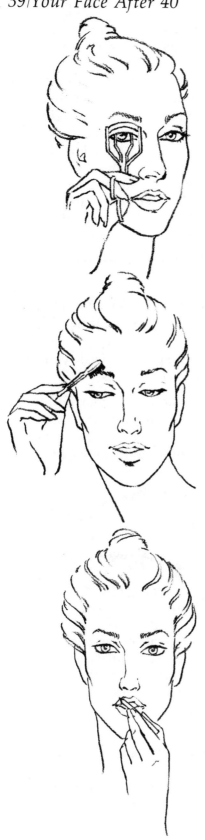

Facing Afternoon

(stronger light, stronger makeup—now you need more definition and color on your face, but textures stay sheer and matte):

• Repowder any shiny spots; whisk away excess. Your face should look fresh, not masky.

• Retouch blusher and lip color.

• Outline the shape of your eye with a gray, blue-gray, gray-green, brown, or mauve pencil. Smudge the line with your finger or an eyeliner brush so it is only a suggestion of a line.

• Add shadow—a color that complements but does not match what you are wearing—with a brush or sponge applicator, over the eye crease, emphasizing outer corners, then under the eye with a thin brush. Blend with fingertips or a wedge of sponge, feathering edges.

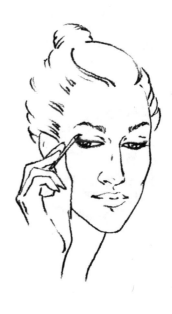

• Add another coat of mascara. Brush brows.

Facing Evening

(time for a complete change and brighter tints of color):

• Cleanse and moisturize your face.

• Apply concealing cream as you did in the morning, then foundation in a formulation slightly more opaque and one shade lighter than your day makeup.

• Powder thoroughly; face should be matte.

• Blusher can be brighter, rosier. Rex often powders the edges of blusher to soften and blend them. Bring blusher lightly over your temples, hairline, and chin.

• Eyes: accentuate them in higher-voltage colors. Rim inner lower lashline with pale blue pencil, then outline upper and lower lashlines with a colored pencil, lifting corners slightly. Use a paler shadow on the lid, a brighter shade over the crease and at the outer eye corners, bringing it under the eye as well. Blend lines to a blur. Add a dab of highlighter under the center of the brow to pick it up.

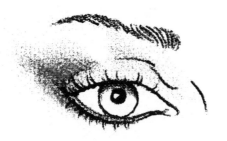

• Curl lashes and apply three to four coats of mascara in navy, violet, deep green, brown, or burgundy. Separate lashes. Fill brows in with pencil and brush them up.

• Outline your lips and fill in with a vibrant lipstick that works with your outfit. Avoid colors that are too blue (they look even bluer), too brown (at night they look like mud), or too yellow (they make teeth look yellow). Finish with a dot of gloss in the center of the lower lip. Blot.

FIVE FAST WAYS TO BRING OUT YOUR EYES

For these special effects you may need special products.

1. Line the top of your lid with a gold eye pencil—keep the line a thin sliver, close to lashes, from the inner eye corner to the outer edge.

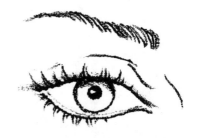

2. For greatest impact, select shadow in shades that *contrast* with your eye color—those that match do not emphasize enough. Eye-catching combinations include:

Blue eyes—shadows in mauve-heather, rust-amber
Gray eyes—shadows in lavenders, teals, midblue to navy

Brown eyes—shadows in peach-amber, mauve-heather, teals
Green eyes—shadows in mauve-heather, midblue to navy, coppers, grays

3. Shade your lid with a light neutral hue—pale brown, taupe, heather, gray—then rim the inner upper and lower lashlines with white pencil. Line the outer lower lashline in soft gray or taupe pencil. Finish with gray or brown mascara on curled upper and lower lashes.

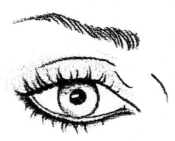

4. Color the eyelid with a pale matte gray or taupe shadow. Bring a deep hue over the crease, beginning about one-quarter inch from inner eye corner. Extend shadow out, then up toward the brow. Line this color under the eye with a thin brush from the center of the lower lid, out at corner and up toward the brow. Blend colors into each other so there are no edges. Mascara upper lashes only.

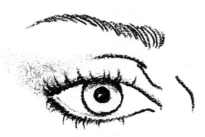

5. Cover the entire eye area from upper lashline to brow in a flat matte brown or gray shadow. Smooth a bit of highlighter under the center portion of the brow. Using a soft dark gray, brown, or gray-blue pencil, follow the lower lashline from the center of the eye to outer corner, lifting corner up; line the outer corner of the upper lashline. Smudge the lines with your finger or an eyeliner brush. Curl lashes and apply mascara to upper lashes only.

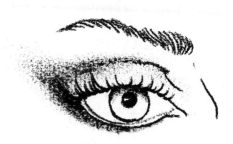

MAKEUP AFTER PLASTIC SURGERY

"If it's true that the surgical procedure turned the clock back ten years, then it is also true that you cannot return to the same hair and makeup you wore before surgery. You probably now need a lighter hand," offers Pablo Manzoni, a leading beauty expert and consultant, formerly with Elizabeth Arden. "Before, your lipstick might have been heavier because your jowls were, so now consider a sheerer lipstick, even a tinted gloss. Before, you may have needed much more shadow and mascara because of puffiness and circles; now, do less—it will say more!"

Test yourself. After surgery, put your makeup on the way you had been wearing it, then examine your face objectively in the mirror. Does Pablo's advice apply to you? Even if it does not, try making just one change—foundation texture or color, blusher placement, lipstick outline. Think simplification and notice the difference it makes.

PROBLEM-SOLVING WITH MAKEUP

"Perfection is so boring that it makes me yawn," says Pablo. "The greatest beauties in this world have marvelous little imperfections for which they are remembered. You have to be a little different or you are confused in the crowd. I like Lauren Hutton; her features are a little crooked, she is unique, imperfect, memorable. Look at Sophia Loren—she's over forty-five and quite remarkable."

Impact comes with individualism, at this stage of life particularly—making the most of the something special *you* have to offer. And isn't it a relief not to have to try to look perfect? There are, however, certain imperfections that come with age for which you may not want to be remembered. Don't despair; these call for the judicious use of corrective camouflage:

Age spots

Often a result of oversunning, these brown areas can be covered by cream concealer applied under your foundation. If your spots are raised or too numerous to conceal in this manner, speak to your dermatolo-gist and in the meantime emphasize your best features to draw attention *away* from imperfections.

Blemishes

Breakouts can occur at every age! Hide, while you heal, a trouble spot with medicated flesh-tinted cream or stick, dotted over the blemish, under your foundation.

Broken blood vessels, birthmarks, scars

Blood vessels can often be covered with concealer, then foundation. If marks are too pronounced, try Covermark by Lydia O'Leary, an opaque makeup created to camouflage serious skin problems. It is available in cream or stick form.

Crepey eyelids

The thin skin of the eyelids loses elasticity very quickly, often appearing wrinkled and old while the rest of your face is still firm and trim. Make lids look smoother with flat matte eye shadow in a subtle neutral shade—taupe, gray, brown, gray-blue. Shiny, frosted, and pearled formulations play up every crease, just what you want to avoid.

Crow's-feet

These lines that collect at the outer corners of the eyes are the signs of facial expression and can't be concealed with makeup because it will crack and crease. They can, however, be softened with cream, smoothed on after you cleanse your face. Wait several minutes for the cream (either a rich moisturizer or undereye cream) to be absorbed, then gently blot off excess with a tissue. Sponge on your foundation and proceed with your makeup. Consider making your mouth a focal point to draw attention away from lines. A soft frame of hair also plays down crow's-feet—don't wear hair pulled severely back from your face. Crow's-feet can be treated by a plastic surgeon or dermatologist. More about this procedure in Chapter 6.

Droopy underbrows

Stan Place suggests this easy trick to make the eye area look smoother and tauter and to minimize fleshiness under the brow: apply a thin layer of brown cream eye shadow over the entire eyelid from the upper lashline to the eyebrow. With a wedge of sponge or your finger, blend it so totally that it merely darkens the skin, then brush a neutral powder shadow over the lid only.

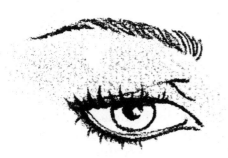

Drooping mouth corners

When the outer lip corners begin to relax, the mouth looks droopy and dour. Start by lightening the folds around the mouth with concealer and blend edges well. Spread foun-

dation over all, including the lips; with a lip pencil outline the upper lip, bringing the line just inside the natural corners. Extend the bottom lipline, lifting it up slightly in each corner. Fill in with color.

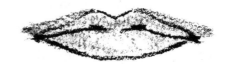

Drooping nose tip

A by-product of advancing years, a drooping nose can be visually corrected with subtle contouring, says makeup expert Emily Pattner. She uses a light brown matte powder eye shadow and a sponge-tip applicator to work her magic: after she applies foundation and face powder, she softens the end of the nose with shadow, smoothing it lightly from the tip to the base of the nostrils. She blends thoroughly with her fingertip, softening the edges until there is a barely perceptible shadow, then retouches the nose with translucent face powder. She checks the final effect in daylight to make sure it is not noticeable. "Barely there" are key words.

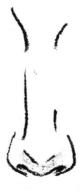

Fleshy jowls and chin

Emily Pattner practices corrective contouring on these relaxed areas as well, but again cautions that it has to be practically invisible to be effective. She starts with a contour powder in a cool, flat brown, applied after foundation and face powder. With a special contour brush, one with short, angled bristles, she tones down the jowls by sweeping contour powder along the jawline from the earlobe to the center of the chin, then from the opposite earlobe, again to the center of the chin. For a double chin she covers the entire area from chin to the top of the throat. She blends and smooths contouring with a cotton ball until it is a faint shadow that she repowders with face powder. Whenever possible she checks the final look in daylight.

Heavy and/or drooping eyebrows

"Thick droopy brows are very aging," explains beauty professional Shelley Durham, who underscores that your goal after forty is to lift your face and features, visually counteracting the gravity that is pulling everything, including the brows, down. "You want a thinner, cleaner, lighter brow with a better defined line to open the face and bring it up."

Brows should be one shade lighter than your hair, unless that color is silver or pale blond, and then they should be more than one shade darker—but always in the same color family. If your brows are too dark, lighten them with facial hair bleach or have them professionally bleached. If they are too light, darken them slightly with brow pencil. Correct and shape your brows in this manner:

• Begin your brow where a pencil lined up against your nostril and over the tear duct of your eye intersects it. Place a dot here as a guide.

• End your brow where the pencil held diagonally across your face, touching the outer part of your nostril and the outer eye corner, intersects the brow. Place a dot here, too.

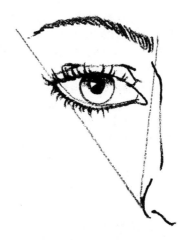

• You want the arch to follow the natural curve of your brow—feel it with your fingertips. Apply dots along it with brow pencil.

• Smudge the dots with your fingertip or brow brush—this will give you a tweezing guideline.

• Keep brows the same width throughout, thinning them gradually and naturally at the ends to give the face a gentle lift.

• Tweeze away excess hair between the brows, and strays that grow outside the curve. If your eye area is easily irritated, desen-

sitize it by rubbing an ice cube over your skin before you tweeze.
• Always tweeze hair under, not over, the brow. If there are any wiry or unruly hairs within the brow that spoil the line, tweeze them out. The curve should be clean, but not perfect, and slightly ragged underneath to look natural.
• Groom brows with a little petroleum jelly on a brush or by brushing them in place, then stroking on a brow fixative.

Lines around the lips

These fine lines cause lipstick to "bleed" and smear. Begin by applying your foundation over your mouth. With a sharpened lip pencil in the same shade as your lipstick, carefully outline lips. If they are too thin, shape them slightly outside the natural line; too thick, keep the line slightly inside the natural curves. Dip a cotton swab into your face

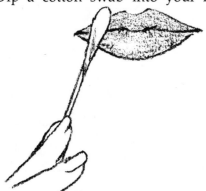

powder and lightly powder this outline. Fill in with lipstick brushed from the center of the lips out to the sides. A creamy formulation is best, in a matte shade. Blot lips gently. If they look dry, apply a sheer dot of a clear gloss in the center of the lower lip. Blot lightly.

Lines from nose to outer mouth corners

These, the nasolabial folds, become more pronounced with age and can be treated surgically (see Chapter 6). You can, however, minimize them in the same manner as undereye pouches by stroking cream concealer over the lines, blending edges with your fingertips or a wedge of sponge, then covering with foundation.

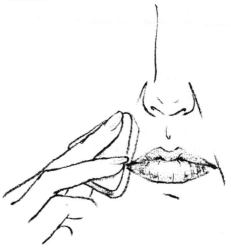

Red-rimmed eyes

If redness is due to irritation, avoid wearing makeup until the condition is cleared. You can offset naturally pink lids by lining the inner rim of the lower lashline with light blue pencil. This will also help the eyes themselves look whiter. Also, prime your upper lid with flesh-colored eye-shadow base; it offsets redness, keeps shadow on longer.

Thin, pale eyelashes

Like your hair, your lashes have a tendency to thin slightly now. If they are light as well, have them professionally dyed to provide a dark underbase for mascara. With a soft black pencil, rim the inner upper lashline, then curl lashes with an eyelash curler and powder them lightly with your translucent face powder. Stroke on mascara. Continue to powder lashes in between successive coats of mascara to build up and thicken them. Always separate lashes with a lash brush or comb.

Undereye bags and pouches

Emily Pattner first places damp, chilled tea bags over the eyes to reduce swelling. Lie on your back with your head propped up, close your eyes and keep tea bags over them for fifteen minutes. Then, with an eyeliner brush, "paint" concealer into the darkest part of the indentation around the pouch and pat-press it with your ring finger (it exerts the least amount of pressure), keeping the concentration of concealer in the indentation. Feather out the edges with fingertips or a wedge of dampened sponge, then apply foundation.

Washed-out skin tone

Skin loses pigment with the years, but you can bring back the bloom with blusher. Select a fresh, clear color—coral, rose, apricot—in powder form, which is easiest to place and blend. With a blusher brush, apply color high on the cheekbone and sweep it up toward the hairline, curving it softly around the temple. With a wedge of sponge, blend it to a whisper.

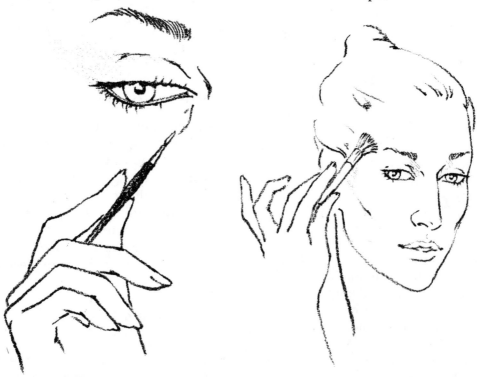

EYEGLASSES—THE NEW COSMETIC

Beauty accessory, beauty necessity. Today's glasses are indispensable beauty helpers—instant eye and cheek makeup, as well as clever problem-area concealers, allowing you to see the world from a vantage point. "I like them quite light and large, never heavy, so they look like you chose them out of desire, rather than need—even if you can't see an inch without them," comments Pablo. "Glasses are marvelous for masking a bit, creating a shield when you are tired. A tinted lens, darker at the top and lighter underneath, also counteracts the dark circles that everyone over twenty-one has!"

Whether you wear them to see or be seen in, to slip over contact lenses or over tired eyes, eyewear has never looked better—you'll find special frames, lenses, and colors for all reasons. "And eyewear, like makeup, should work with face shape and skin tone, hair color and style, wardrobe, and most important, personality," stresses Stephan Laudicino, vice-president of Lugene Opticians, an exclusive eyewear boutique that offers new designs every two months.

Glasses as makeup

"If a woman thought of eyewear in the same way she does a scarf or a shoe, as an accessory that enhances and completes her look, she wouldn't have difficulty with selection," explains Laudicino. "Just as the same pair of shoes won't work with every outfit, neither will the same pair of glasses. You'll probably need at least two pairs to start—one for casual wear and the other for more formal attire, and both to complement the most important colors in your day or evening wardrobes. And throw out those rules about certain frames for certain face shapes—you have to experiment with eyewear, and try on frames until you find those that do what you want them to and are true to your style." To help you put your choice in the proper perspective, our expert offers these general guidelines:

• Frames should work with your face shape *and* height *and* body type—always try them on in front of a full-length mirror.
• The ideal frame accentuates every good point in the face.

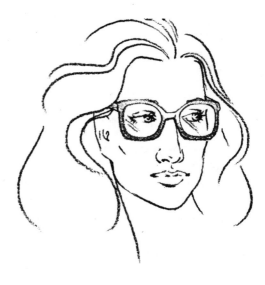

• Those with an upward curve in the top corners "lift" the features, offsetting relaxed facial contours.
• The placement of the temple bar

can also solve problems—a high bar visually raises the face; a center bar detracts from the thickness of the lens; a low bar can help to hide crow's-feet and facial lines.

• A high bridge adds length to the nose, while a more centrally located one will shorten the nose.

• Hairstyle influences frame size and shape—don't buy glasses the

imizing the prescription and camouflaging lines and wrinkles.

• Think gradient frames to correct facial flaws: a clear bridge deemphasizes the nose; a paler rather than darker top deaccentuates a full forehead, and it adds height to a low forehead.

• Think gradient lenses—always darker on top, lighter at the base:

The following color combinations might be good starting points:

Skin-Hair Color	Complementary Frame Colors
fair/blond	pastels: blue, violet, beige; pale tortoiseshell, gold
fair/light brown	muted blues, beiges, reds; peach; tortoiseshell, gold, bronze
fair/brunette	brights: red, blue; copper; wine
sallow/any color	warm shades of peach, red, amber, pink; midblues. Avoid yellow, green
ruddy/any color	cool shades of blue or green; wine; gold, silver. Avoid violets, taupes, rose
any color/gray	lilacs, pale blues, pinks, silver, aquas. Avoid yellow, transparents
fair/red	cool shades of blue and green; wine; tortoiseshell, gold, brown, beige

day before you are making a hair change.

• Consider wardrobe color along with natural coloring. Like anything else you put on, eyewear should complement your coloring, not overpower it. Soft, subtle tints are generally most flattering, but brights can give your face an attractive color boost.

• The frame and lens tints should harmonize—tinted lenses are fashionable and effective for not only enhancing the eyes but min-

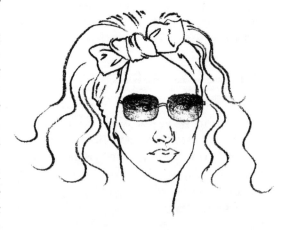

blue brightens away tiredness; a blush-toned bottom adds glow and a healthy wash of color to pale skin, livens sallowness, too; a honey or peach tone at bottom neutralizes reddened eyelids.

• Consider the ornamental value of frames. If you need reading glasses, let them be conversation pieces: an antique or modern lorgnette, half glasses in exciting colors that fold to slip in your purse.

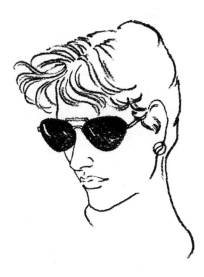

• Remember the protective value of dark sunglasses—they are vital in sun, wind, and pollution, plus they cut down on aging squint lines. Best lens colors for screening out light without distortion are gray, deep green, and brown—the brighter the light, the darker you want your lens to be. If you are sensitive to glare, consider polarized lenses. Photochromatic lenses adjust to the light level—lighten indoors and darken outdoors. However, they never darken sufficiently to offer the best sun protection.

Makeup for glasses

"With tinted lenses especially, you can wear more eye makeup," says Pablo. "The same if you are nearsighted and lenses are thick, since anything behind them disappears 20 percent." But there is a fine line between more and too much more. Keep the following in mind when you are making up:

• If your glasses cast a shadow or make your eyes look smaller, add more makeup, but in soft, gentle shades—anything too dark will close up the eye.

• If your lenses magnify your eyes, you may need less makeup but more thoroughly blended—every lash separated—because all flaws are accentuated.

• A tinted lens can change the eye makeup shade underneath it. Check the finished look in daylight with your glasses on.

• Oversized tinted lenses can change your cheek color too. You may need less color since a blush-hued lens over a blushed cheek could look overdone. Your lipstick should then harmonize with your glasses as well.

About your eyesight

Have you noticed that you are suddenly having more difficulty seeing close up now and have to hold the newspaper, a book, or a menu farther away from your face? This decline in the ability to focus—a natural part of the eye's aging process, is known as presbyopia, and it happens to everyone. "It doesn't start when you're forty," explains Dr. Robert Maynard, a Phoenix optometrist and chairman of the Communications Division of the American Optometric Association. "It just starts to become a problem at about this age. Near vision actually begins to deteriorate at age ten and continues gradually throughout life. At the same time that the lens of the eye becomes less elastic, the eye muscle ceases to expand and contract efficiently, so that the lens becomes more fixed and focus is affected. Nearsighted people might even find reading more comfortable without their glasses."

Reading glasses or bifocal or trifocal lenses easily correct presbyopia. Newest of the multifocals are no-line lenses, which fall into two basic types: the first contains an invisible seam between the near and the far vision segments. The second, known as a progressive addition lens, has powers that increase gradually from the distance to the near vision segment. By moving your head, you can insure clear vision at all distances. Contact lenses, too, offer a viable alternative to glasses for correcting presbyopia, says Dr. Maynard, and there is a range of lens designs and fitting techniques your doctor can choose from.

Contact lenses

Whether for vanity or sharper sight—contact lenses provide more accurate and natural vision than glasses because they are so close to the eye and move with it, allowing you always to look through the center of the lens where vision is best—the percentage of Americans wearing contact lenses has more than tri-

pled in the last decade, estimates the American Optometric Association. Seventy-one percent of all wearers are female, 46 percent of them are twenty-five to forty-four years old, and 14 percent are forty-five or older. And, due to advances in lens design, materials, prescription, and fit that makes them more appealing and useful to an older segment of the population, there are indications that the size of this latter segment will be growing.

The two major categories of lenses are hard and soft. The newest hard lens is gas permeable, composed of a combination of the standard hard plastic and silicone; it is larger and thinner than the standard lens. Soft lenses are available in a variety of types, including the new extended-wear lenses. While they differ in chemical composition, they are all fabricated of some form of liquid-absorbing plastic, which renders them flexible when wet to conform to the surface of the eye.

Best for correcting presbyopia are:
• bifocal contact lenses—these are hard and take some getting used to. They do, however, allow comfortable vision at all seeing distances.
• a contact lens for one eye only—prescribed for reading only, and a satisfactory solution for some people.
• single vision contact lenses—these correct distance vision but you still need reading glasses to correct near vision.
• monovision—this treatment is for someone who has good vision in both eyes and does not favor

one eye over the other. As Dr. Maynard explains, one eye is fitted with a contact lens for distance vision and the other eye is fitted for near vision. While depth perception can be slightly affected, it is in no way handicapped.

Makeup for contact lenses

• Remove any hand lotion or cream from the fingers before handling contact lenses
• Insert them before applying makeup
• Do not line the inner rims of the eyelashes—makeup can film lenses
• Use a water-soluble mascara; one with a lash-building formulation can deposit unwanted—and irritating—fibers in your eye
• Powder eye shadow can flake, so do not bring it close to the eye—use a pencil or crayon
• Always remove lenses before cleansing off eye makeup

Chapter 5

Face Care: What You Can Do

Face the world without makeup—you'd never dream of it! But consider how much magic is wasted if the skin beneath your foundation and blusher is not at its fittest. Sheer subtle makeup, which is the way you want to wear it now, can be only as beautiful as the skin it's on. And to keep yours healthy and bright, you have to care for it, but in a, perhaps, new-for-you way—with a program that treats your complexion the way it needs to be treated each day, a program adjusted to the day's weather, activity, the environment, as well as to skin changes. And this program probably won't be the same as it was last year, or even last month. If it is, your skin might not look as good as it could. "Proper skin care has to be balanced and variable—for the season, your life-style and the site of the skin, since skin is not the same all over the face. It's this variability that must be taken into account if you're trying to make skin look better and better," explains Dr. Norman Orentreich, clinical associate professor of dermatology, New York University Medical Center, and director of the Orentreich Foundation for the Advancement of Science.

Yes, your skin is changing, whether noticeably or imperceptibly. Part of this change is inevitable, predetermined by heredity, but a large part of it is avoidable. External factors like sun exposure, low humidity, cold, wind, and smoking age skin prematurely. You'll learn more about them, and how you can control or prevent their effects, in Chapter 7. Here the emphasis is on caring for your skin today—in an easy and uncomplicated way—to improve its appearance and its behavior.

Why is your complexion acting the way it is? Let's peel back the layers for an in-depth look.

YOUR SKIN SIMPLIFIED

Your skin is your largest organ (it makes up about one tenth of your weight), your only visible one, and a good gauge of your health and mood. It can, however, look older—or younger—than its years. The two principal layers that compose it rest on a third, the adipose, or fat, layer, which gives your face its rounded contours. The epidermis, or outer layer, acts as a barrier for the inner layer, the dermis, which provides support and nourishment, including moisture—the vital skin element.

Working from the inside out: the dermis is made up entirely of living tissue. It contains the oil and sweat glands (which empty onto the skin's surface via the pores), hair follicles, blood vessels, and collagen and elastin fibers responsible for skin's elasticity and resiliency. But time brings transformations:

• The collagen and elastin fibers degenerate and lose elasticity and suppleness. The skin toughens and thins owing to a loss of gel-like "ground substance" between fiber bundles. The layer over them—the epidermis—deprived of its resilient support, wrinkles and sags. This process is hastened by exposure to the sun: ultraviolet rays break down collagen fibers, causing them to frazzle faster.

• The flow of the blood through the vessels gives skin its healthy pink glow, but gradually circulation slows down, so that skin loses rosiness. When this happens, cell efficiency is impaired because the blood also transports nutrients and moisture and eliminates toxins. The blood vessels are more easily damaged.

• Moisture is the ingredient that keeps skin soft and smooth; however, the natural supply eventually decreases with aging, which is one of the reasons why skin becomes drier. The oil glands that lock in this moisture, allowing the skin to hold on to the water it needs to stay in shape, reduce production. Deprived of its protective coating, the water already present evaporates more readily. (Sometimes, though, oil glands remain active or speed up their activity, so that skin stays oily or gets even oilier.)

While changes in the dermal layer affect the way your skin looks and acts, those in the outer layer are of course much more apparent. The epidermis is composed of about thirty thin layers that renew themselves over a monthly cycle. Each day dead cells of the outermost surface are shed as new living cells are formed by the base and fed by the dermis. These eventually are pushed up to the surface where they are shed. As you grow older, this process, called the "epidermal turnover time," slows down, new cells are not formed as rapidly, and dead cells stay in place longer, so that the skin's appearance changes—it looks cloudy, coarse, and dull. Living cells lose their plumpness, while the dead ones curl up instead of lying flat, making skin feel rough. This problem is compounded when the atmosphere is dry, so that moisture at the skin's surface evaporates more quickly than it's replaced.

Another change occurs in the color of the skin—the pigment cells, normally evenly distributed, become increasingly uneven, so that skin becomes blotchy—some areas darken, forming brown spots, while others grow paler.

Knowing how and why skin changes occur should help you understand how much you can do about them. You can avoid added problems in the dermis with sunscreens and -blocks. "You need protection against sunlight to prevent damage in the deeper layer of the tissues, damage that shows up ten, fifteen, twenty years later as a wrinkle, brown spot, or little skin cancer," says Dr. Orentreich. To correct surface problems and give your skin the best care on a daily basis, he suggests *exfoliation* and *emolliation*.

THE CONCEPT OF EXFOLIATION/ EMOLLIATION

Exfoliation includes all the techniques to remove the dead surface-cell layer, from the mildest cleansing to the most abrasive sloughing with grains, scrubs, or a nonmedicated cleansing sponge. While not all dermatologists agree upon the necessity of abrasive exfoliation (also known as "epidermabrasion"), there are growing numbers, perhaps foremost among them Dr. Orentreich, who advise making it part of your regular skin-care program. "The rubbing action involved in epidermabrasion actually speeds up epidermal turnover time," he explains, "bringing it back to a younger level of function." He continues, "Cleansing and toning are really two words for the one concept of exfoliation. They are removal techniques that improve the surface texture of the skin. But while they can provide sufficient stimulation for some skins, they are not enough for most skins after forty, when the cell replacement rate has significantly slowed down, and more stimulation is needed." You can find it in the Buf-Puf, the gently abrasive sponge that Dr. Orentreich originally developed to improve the skin surface and texture. It's used with your cleanser—soap, lotion, or cream—to polish your skin to a better cosmetic appearance, a smoother, more translucent state. "You should

carry epidermabrasion to the point where you are aware that something is happening, but short of irritation. You want fresher skin, not irritated skin," he advises. You achieve this by controlling the sponge variables—pressure, speed, and length of time—as well as frequency of use. He adds that the Buf-Puf is not for all complexions—those that are superdelicate and ultradry might be too easily irritated. "But I have no objection to any of the other methods of exfoliation, as long as a woman understands the basic concept—that it improves the texture of the skin. And in order to do this, exfoliation has to be optimal: as much as can be tolerated short of irritation. When it's optimal, she'll also need an emollient—the right moisturizer—to replace the protective oils that have been buffed away."

While the process of exfoliation/emolliation stays the same for every skin, you build variability into your skin-care program through the products you use and their frequency of use. Your skin is as individual as your fingerprint, and no two are exactly alike. However, to provide a starting point for selecting the products that will work best, all skins can be categorized into three general types—dry, normal, and oily—plus a subtype—sensitive.

TESTING YOUR SKIN'S VITAL SIGNS

Dr. Orentreich suggests examining your skin's vital signs in the same way he does: by looking at hair and eye color and response to the sun and wind. Other factors influencing skin are weather, life-style, the environment, heredity—and skin conditions. "Most people are unaware of subliminal dermatoses," he explains, "but they could be the cause of a persistent problem—skin that is perceived as dry, for example. That's why a dermatologist looks not only at the face, but also at the scalp to see if it's scaly; the elbows, to determine if they are rough, and if there are cracks in the skin. There are some dry skins that moisturizing alone cannot correct . . . an appropriate medication is needed to get rid of the underlying cause." While there may be no condition causing your skin to behave the way it does, you may want to keep this possibility in mind if your skin does not respond to the improved care you give it.

Test your skin and its reactions by asking yourself the following questions:

1. What type of skin do your parents have?
2. What color are your eyes?
3. What's the natural color of your hair?
4. How does your skin feel?
5. Is your skin light, medium, or dark?
6. Can you see your pores?
7. Do you have blackheads? Breakouts?
8. Does your skin look shiny? Where?
9. How does your skin react to wind?
10. Does your skin redden and chap easily?
11. Do you burn in the sun?
12. Do you have lines and wrinkles?
13. Is your skin flaky?

Note your response on a piece of paper to determine a profile of your skin type, then compare it with those that follow. You may not neatly fit into one category. Skin differs over the face, as well as season to season—so that the same face parched by January cold might be moist and shiny in July. Most skin, however, say the experts, is normal, although not all normal skins are alike—and most grow drier with age.

Dry skin

Your skin is *probably*—but not necessarily—dry if it is very fair and you have light hair and eyes, or dark hair with light skin and eyes. Your mother probably has dry skin, and this profile of skin characteristics applies to you as well:
   • skin always burns in the sun
   • pores are very small
   • even texture, flat finish—skin may look flaky and dull
   • skin feels dry and chapped
   • skin sometimes gets so raw and dry that it cracks
   • tendency toward crinkly lines and wrinkles
   • skin probably blemish-free

Normal skin

Your skin is *probably* normal if it's fair and your eyes are not too light; your hair may be light, medium, or dark. Your parents both probably have normal skin. Other skin characteristics include:

- skin usually burns a little before tanning
- pores are small and fairly uniform in size, larger around the nose
- smooth, even texture
- good balance of oil and moisture—makeup lasts well without caking or showing oily breakthrough
- skin may chap in the wind, but moisturizing brings it quickly back to normal
- some expression lines and wrinkles
- skin usually blemish- and blackhead-free

Oily skin

Your skin is *probably* oily if it is olive or sallow and you have dark eyes and hair. You could also be a mixture of types. But your skin has a good oil supply; your parents' skin probably did as well. Other skin characteristics include:

- skin that tans easily without burning
- larger pores
- coarse texture
- shiny skin, especially in the T-zone: forehead, nose, and chin
- skin not adversely affected by wind
- the possibility of acne in adolescence; tendency to blackheads, breakouts

Your skin—whether it's dry, normal, or oily—might also be sensitive, easily irritated. Characteristics of sensitive skin are:

- a thin surface layer
- splotchiness—patches of red
- inability to tolerate fragrance, alcohol, the sun and wind, anything abrasive
- fragility—it's vulnerable and probably marked by tiny broken capillaries

Many cosmetic companies have taken the guesswork out of treatment selection by grouping formulations according to skin needs—normal, oily, dry, sensitive—and some according to age. However, those aimed at mature skin are usually heavily moisturized—fine if skin is dry, but not suitable if it's oily, except on a special-occasion basis, when skin is overexposed to the elements and temporarily dried out.

YOUR SKIN-CARE STRATEGY

Following are the essentials of daily and special care for your skin, with ways to beat the heat, sun, cold, and wind. Remember, if your skin is a combination, treat each area the way it needs treating: with the right formulations.

Dry skin
Every Day
- Morning: Cleanse with a neutral or nondetergent soap if skin can't tolerate soap; or a cleansing cream or lotion, alternated occasionally with soap. Follow with at least three rinsings of warm water to remove all traces of soap or cleanser. Smooth moisturizer over skin while it's still damp. Protect the thin and fragile skin under

your eyes with an eye cream, dotted on from outer eye corner to inner. After ten minutes blot excess with a tissue.

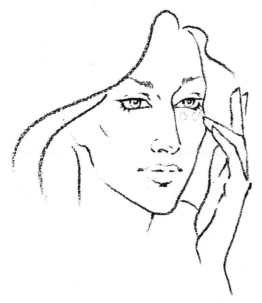

• Evening: Gently remove eye makeup with a cream, lotion, or oil remover and a tissue, so that you do not have to tug on this fragile area. Cleanse as you did in the morning, then apply toner with a cotton pad, and sweep a thin layer of night cream over your face and throat to moisturize skin while you sleep.

Special Care

• Once or twice a week, depending on your skin's dryness and sensitivity, brighten your complexion by sloughing off dead-skin buildup with an abrasive scrub or sponge. Keep pressure light and build time gradually. Always follow with a film of moisturizer.
• Once a week, follow cleansing with a rich moisturizing mask to smooth and soften skin.

Weather/Environment

• Cold, windy weather draws moisture from the skin and causes it to chap. Always keep skin lubricated with enriched formulations before you go outdoors. Add more moisture to your environment with plants and a cold-mist vaporizer.
• Overexposure to the sun is particularly devastating, since dry skin burns so easily. Protect with a high sun protection factor (SPF) sunscreen, sunscreen-formulated makeups, too.
• Skin stays moister when air is warm and humid, but feels dirtier, as perspiration does not evaporate quickly. Cleanse skin meticulously, cool and refresh it with a nonalcohol toner, change your moisturizer to a lighter formulation. Your skin may need more frequent exfoliation: build up to it slowly.
(*Note:* Air conditioning is very drying. If you are continually in an air-conditioned environment, you have to step up your moisturizing and add more moisture to the air with plants or a vaporizer.)

Normal skin

Every Day

• Morning: Cleanse with a mild soap and rinse skin thoroughly with at least three changes of warm water to remove any soap residue, which can be irritating. Over your still-damp skin smooth a sheer moisturizer wherever skin feels dry and taut. Then protect the delicate skin of your under-eyes by dotting an eye cream from

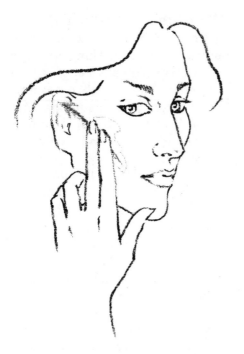

outer eye corner to inner. After ten minutes blot excess with tissue.

• Evening: Remove eye makeup gently with a cream, lotion, or oil remover and a tissue, then cleanse your face as you did in the morning. Use a toner on oilier areas if you feel you need it, then apply night cream on dry areas only.

Special Care

• At least twice a week, more often if your skin can tolerate it, slough off cellular buildup with an abrasive scrub or sponge, concentrating on oilier areas. Always follow with a moisturizer.

• Once a week, moisturize your skin with a refreshing, moisturizing mask, smoothed onto your throat as well.

Weather/Environment

• Windy winter weather is drying. Protect your skin with a richer moisturizer when you go out-

doors; cream the throat as well as the eye area, since they both are particularly sensitive to the drying effects of cold and wind. Soap should be more emollient, and if you find soap too drying, alternate it with a nonsoap or cleansing lotion. Exfoliate less frequently and/or moisturize more if skin is chapped and dry.

• In summer your skin needs a sunscreen for protection, and possibly a moisturizer to seal in moisture that the sun's heat outdoors—and air conditioning indoors—can evaporate. Warm, humid air may make your T-zone especially shiny, and since oily areas get dirty faster, cleanse your face thoroughly and exfoliate more frequently with an abrasive surface, paying special attention to oilier areas. Sweep off excess oils with a toner containing some alcohol. Moisturize dry areas only.

Oily skin

Every Day

• Morning: Wash with soap and an abrasive cleansing sponge that whisks off dead skin and any

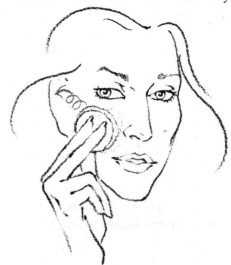

dulling film. Pat skin dry and apply a water-based moisturizer to any dry areas, and a richer cream over the undereye area, which is usually dry because there are fewer oil glands. Dot a film of cream from outer eye corner to inner and after 10 minutes, blot excess with a tissue.

• Evening: Remove eye makeup with an oil, cream, or lotion remover, then wash your face with soap, rinsing it with at least three changes of warm water to remove any irritating traces of soap. If your T-zone is especially oily, saturate a cotton pad with toner and sweep it over this area. And if your skin is especially oily, use your abrasive sponge in the evenings as well.

Special Care

• Control any oil breakthrough during the day with astringent or toner on a cotton pad. If that is too drying, just dampen the cotton pad or try a linen blotting tissue—it won't disturb your makeup either.

• Once a week, use a clay mask to deep-cleanse the skin and boost its glow.

• Dry up breakouts with a cream, or lotion with a benzoyl peroxide base, dabbed over them.

Weather/Environment

• Cold, windy weather is less likely to chap oily skin since it has a natural layer of protection, but it will nonetheless feel drier in cold weather. You may want to switch to a milder soap and toner and cleanse with an abrasive sponge every other day. Moisturize dry areas and protect the drier throat and undereyes with cream.

• Hot, humid weather appears to speed up the activity of the oil glands—skin gets dirtier as more oil is emulsified by perspiration. Cleanse scrupulously and epidermabrade the skin daily to keep it fresh and unclogged. Absorb excess oil with a toner or blotting linen during the day, and if you wish, follow with a dusting of face powder to cut down shine and keep face matte. If air conditioning is dehydrating the skin, reduce epidermabrasion or use of toner or increase moisturizing dry areas, preferably while they are slightly damp. Add more moisture to your surroundings with plants or a vaporizer.

Sensitive skin

Sensitive skin, whether it's dry, normal, or oily, needs gentle bland care with nonirritating, fragrance-free products. Cleanse with a neutral soap, a nonsoap, or a nonfragranced cream or lotion, depending upon skin type. Rinse with warm water at least three times to remove any potentially irritating residue. Moisturize dry areas only, including the undereye area. If skin is too delicate to exfoliate with an abrasive scrub or sponge, try a washcloth. Alternate this with an alcohol-free freshener on oily areas in particular, and a weekly mask—a moisturizing one on dry skin, a clay-based mask on oily skin.

Lessen the risk of broken capillaries, to which sensitive skin is prone, by avoiding extreme heat and cold,

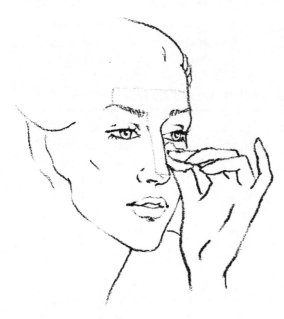

for eyes and throat. Your skin will need a variety of formulations, depending upon the external stresses it is up against.

Exfoliators

These sweep away dirt, makeup, pollutants, cellular debris, and excess oils that make skin look coarser, thicker, older; they allow for easier hydration so that skin looks plumper, feels smoother.

• *Makeup removers*—creams, lotions, or oils that dissolve makeup, particularly mascara, so that you can gently tissue them off, a job that soaps and ordinary cleansers cannot perform as efficiently. Apply the remover with

massage and rough handling, and drinking alcohol in excess.

Protect your sensitive skin from the sun in summer, with a sunscreen or -block—in makeups as well. In winter protect with moisturizers; always dress warmly and cover the lower part of your face as much as possible with a scarf or muffler.

WHAT TO EXPECT FROM YOUR SKIN-CARE PREPARATIONS

Following Dr. Orentreich's guideline, all treatment products can be slotted into two categories: *exfoliators*, which improve the surface texture of the skin—they include makeup removers, cleansers, toners, masks, and sloughers—and *emollients*, which soothe and smooth skin, trapping its vital moisture—they include moisturizers, night creams, and special purpose creams

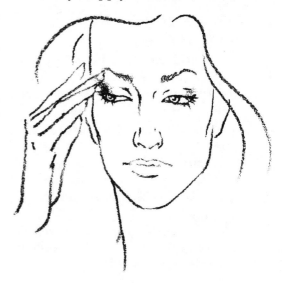

your fingertips or a cotton swab, massage lightly, tissue off. Then wash your face.

• *Cleansers*—clean off stale makeup, excess oils, dirt, cellular debris. *Soap* is the most efficient cleanser but may not be gentle enough for every skin. Says Dr. Orentreich, "I'm very much for frequent washing, but I'm not for using soap when you're irritated and dry."

Soap is generally better for normal and oily skins; dry and sensitive types are less likely to be irritated by cream or lotion cleansers, or mild nonsoaps. However, there is virtually a soap or soap-based product for every skin some of the time—Dove or Neutrogena for dry, sensitive skin, a lower pH soap, oatmeal, or Lowila Cake soap, just to name a few, for normal or even oily skin. They can be alternated with cream or lotion cleansers whenever skin is too dry.

The correct way to cleanse is first to wet your face with warm or tepid water, then work up a soapy lather in your hands, quickly massage it lightly over your face and jawline.

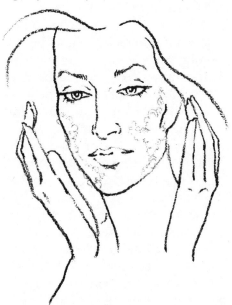

Rinse at least three times with warm water to remove any residue, then pat skin dry.

• *Cleansing creams and lotions*—are not as drying as soap, although many contain some kind of soap. They should be massaged into the skin according to individual directions, then either tissued off or rinsed directly off with water. Creams are usually richer than lotions; lotions contain the same ingredients but with a higher percentage of water.

• *Toners, fresheners, astringents*—continue the cleansing process by removing soap or cleanser residue, oil, and any other surface debris still on the skin after cleansing. Alcohol is usually the active ingredient in all of these products—it makes skin feel fresh and cool because it evaporates quickly, and it temporarily minimizes pores by plumping up the skin around them. The percentage of alcohol differs from product to product, and the words toner, freshener, and astringent are more or less interchangeable. Water-based toners and fresheners are formulated especially for those skins that cannot tolerate alcohol. Apply by dampening a cotton pad with toner and sweeping it over the face until it comes away clean. Toning is a good way to refresh the skin during the day in hot sticky weather.

• *Masks*—are usually cleansers and/or oil absorbers; they take many of the loose surface cells with them when they are removed. Their tightening action can boost circulation, and some masks form a watertight shield that permits a moisture buildup underneath. Gel-type masks are better for normal and dry skins, while clay masks help oily skins.

If you have combination skin—oily in the center and dry at the edges—use a clay mask over oily areas and a moisturizing mask everywhere else.

There are many masks you can make yourself that provide a quick pickup. These are from Lydia Sarfati of the Klisar Skin Care Center in New York City:

• For dry skin—the egg-yolk and honey mask softens and nourishes: mix one egg yolk with one teaspoon honey to a smooth consistency. Massage your face and throat with a rich cream, then wait seven minutes so that oil glands will be stimulated and ready for the mask. Spread it evenly over the face; leave on for fifteen minutes, then rinse off with warm water. Follow with a moisturizer.

• For dry, sensitive, and chapped skin—the buttermilk soothing mask: leave buttermilk out overnight so that the thick part rises. Pat it gently over the skin. Leave on for fifteen minutes, rinse off. Moisturize.

• For oily skin—a yeast-based mask that tones down shine: mix one packet of yeast with warm water to make a paste. Smooth all over the face. Leave on for ten minutes, then rinse thoroughly with tepid water.

• Sloughers—designed to lift off dead surface cells and speed up cell regeneration. In this category are abrasive creams and grains, and abrasive sponges like the Buf-Puf. They improve skin texture and appearance; clean pores, making them look smaller; and allow moisturizers to work better because the dry, tough outer-cell layer is removed. A sponge can be used with your cleanser of choice and give you as much or as little sloughing action as you wish. It's important that you use the slougher that's right for your skin at the time, and in the right manner. You may have to experiment with several to learn which is best.

Emollients

These are the lubricating creams and lotions that seal in skin's moisture while soothing and softening the epidermis.

• Moisturizers—return some of the oils lost in the exfoliating process. They stay on the skin's surface—some penetrate it slightly—to slow down moisture loss with a protective film. They help to offset tightness and make skin feel more comfortable, while softening fine lines and wrinkles caused by dryness. Moisturizers should only be used where your skin is dry: the formulation you choose depends upon your skin's needs—and if you're exfoliating optimally, you'll need to put back those oils you've taken away.

All moisturizers contain oil, and the thinner the cream, the more water it contains. Water-based products have more water than oil; oil-based products contain more oil than water. You can test the richness of the formulation by applying a little on the back of your hand. If it leaves a high shine, it's oil-based; if it doesn't, it's water-based.

• *Night creams*—are generally heavier than moisturizers. Use them to guard against overnight moisture loss—particularly if a room is overheated or air-conditioned—when your skin is dry. If your skin is normal or a combination of oily and dry, use them on dry areas only.

• *Eye and throat creams*—are rich creams, some containing ingredients to tighten the eye and throat areas while lubricating them. All mature skins regardless of type need the lubricating protection of an eye cream. Throat creams are helpful if you feel that your moisturizer is not rich enough for your thin, ultradry throat skin.

Thanks to medical research there is a range of products that help you help your skin, and there may be more to come. "One of my major research efforts," explains Dr. Orentreich, "is to find a variety of 'messengers' that can be applied to the skin's surface to talk to the hair follicles, oil glands, and collagen, telling them to behave younger. We've already found medicines that will stimulate oil production, but we don't have those that will make collagen and elastin younger—yet. But we're getting there. And this is not skin rejuvenation in an alchemic, magical way—rather, we want to counteract deficiencies where they exist; to attempt to stimulate the body to produce chemicals that it produced at a younger age, at a more rapid pace, to stimulate the skin's own natural functions! Just as epidermabrasion with the Buf-Puf, for example, can revitalize the epidermis, we're searching for means to stimulate the dermis—collagen, elastin."

Varying your daily care to meet skin's changing cycles, to correct its surface problems and speed up its responses so that it will look brighter and fresher—these are the important things you can do for yourself. But sometimes even the best skin because of prior abuse (sun damage takes years to show up) needs professional help. Says Dr. Orentreich, "You yourself can buff and polish your epidermis to a better cosmetic appearance, but when the dermis is sun-damaged, withered and weathered, it needs professional resurfacing—dermabrasion or chemical peeling." Sometimes it also needs to have lost tissues replaced or sagging tissues redraped—and all of these procedures are the provinces of your dermatologist or plastic surgeon.

Chapter 6

Your Face: What a Doctor Can Do

"I like a look of experience—lines around the eyes, a face that appears a little rumpled, sleepy. It makes me think that a woman has been up all night making love," a worldly young Frenchman once confided. Wrinkles *can* be attractive, considered by many to be medals of honor—signs of life, animation, expression. But if you feel that yours are more like battle scars, there are ways of doing away with them. This is where cosmetic medicine can help you face up to the future: plastic surgery, dermatology, cosmetic dentistry. The three often work together; in fact, they sometimes overlap. When do you need them, and what can they do for you?

PLASTIC SURGERY

"Need? Need is subjective. Plastic surgery is a question of desire—to be considered when you don't like the signs of aging. Everyone ages; it's hereditary. It happens at different times for different people. Surgery should only be performed when the aging process has produced enough changes so that you can see a difference—not enough changes and a woman won't benefit; too many, and she won't benefit

enough," explains Dr. Steven Herman, a New York plastic surgeon. "There is a limit to the power of surgery, though. You can expect to look fresher, more relaxed, yes, younger, but not *young*. Plastic surgery can erase some of the ravages of time, but it can't turn back the clock and make you look twenty!"

But often wrinkles are more than skin-deep. Suppose you're bored, restless, and unhappy; life is not as much fun as it used to be; you feel that you have nothing to look forward to. You look to the lines in your face as the reason and decide that plastic surgery is the solution to your problems. Focusing on a correctable fault for all of the dissatisfaction in life is unrealistic, as is believing that plastic surgery will make you look different than you *ever* did before: the results of surgery can never measure up to the expectations. "You should realize that plastic surgery will produce changes that may *secondarily* alter your life—it can make you feel better about yourself because you look better, and may give you the motivation to get in shape, buy a new wardrobe, change your hairstyle. You'll project this new confidence—feel freer, perhaps, to socialize, find the reaction of others different to you because your attitude is different. But more than that, no," cautions Dr. Herman.

Understanding your skin as well as your psyche should also give you a more realistic goal. Basically, skin thins as it ages; connective tissue becomes less resilient as elastic fibers deep within break down, so that the skin no longer bounces back into place. Muscles stretch and fat pads shift, while gravity exerts a steady downward pull. Changes are gradual but progressive—directed by heredity and hastened by abuse (smoking, the sun, harsh handling, factors that you directly control; but more about them in the next chapter)—and permanent. Once they take place, reversal is out of anyone's hands except a plastic surgeon's.

So, you look in the mirror. You don't hate yourself or your life but you do despise the bags under your eyes, the folds from your nose to your mouth, or the relaxed skin around your chin, and you want to know what you can reasonably expect from plastic surgery. Here, then, to begin, is a checklist of the most common signs of facial aging and the best procedures for correcting them:

COMMON SIGNS OF FACIAL AGING AND THEIR SURGICAL SOLUTIONS

Problem	Solution
• Deep lines and furrows on forehead	• Liquid silicone or Zyderm collagen implants by injection—preferred procedures
	• Forehead lift—involves extensive surgery
• Drooping eyebrows	• Forehead lift—preferred procedure
• Heavy upper lids, overhanging skin	• Eye lift—completely correctable
• Pouches, wrinkles, loose skin under eyes	• Eye lift—completely correctable
• Dark undereye circles	• Area will appear lighter if part of darkly pigmented skin is removed during surgery
• Crow's-feet	• Liquid silicone or Zyderm collagen implants by injection
• Frown lines between the eyes	• Liquid silicone or Zyderm collagen implants by injection
• Nasolabial creases from nose to corner of the mouth	• Cannot be completely removed. A face lift will soften them; can be filled in with injections of liquid silicone or collagen
• Relaxed jowls	• Face lift—completely correctable

- Double chin

- Loose skin and folds on neck

- Drooping nose

- Lengthened earlobes

- Fine lines and wrinkles around the mouth

- A chin lift performed with a face lift to remove fatty tissue—completely correctable

- Face lift—completely correctable. If there is profound sagging and vertical bands, a platysma lift in conjunction with the face lift can correct the problem—still controversial

- The nose is often elevated by removing cartilage at tip during a face lift—completely correctable

- Earlobes are frequently shortened during a face lift—completely correctable

- Dermabrasion or chemical peeling gives good results. A face lift cannot remove fine lines. May be some pigment change

Although the charted procedures are listed separately, they are often performed in tandem. The face is not composed of isolated parts, and several areas at a time may need attention to give harmony to the total look. Many doctors feel that the more extensive the face lift, the more natural-looking the outcome, since broad separation of the skin from its underlying facial structures enables it to be redraped without distortion.

It is not uncommon then for a surgeon to elevate the tip of the nose, shorten the earlobes, and peel away the fine lines around the lips at the same time as he does a face lift.

Eye lift

Eyelid surgery can accompany a face lift, but more often will precede it by a number of years. Eyelid skin is thin and loose, unbound to underlying muscles, and in an extremely vulnerable position. It is stretched and pulled whenever you blink, move your eyes, apply makeup or remove it, as well as affected by external forces that etch in lines—the sun, cigarettes, wind. It's no wonder that the eye area ages prematurely, faster than any other on the face!

An eye lift performed by a competent surgeon can whisk away the years, along with the bags, pouches, and crepiness. It is particularly long-lasting because gravity does not pull the lids down as quickly as it does the facial skin. Usually both lids are corrected at the same time, but they can be done independently of each other. The eyes are marked to indicate the amount of skin that has to be removed. A local anesthetic is administered; an incision is made in the crease of the upper eyelid, and excess skin and protruding fat are removed. The skin is closed with tiny sutures. Along the lower lid the incision is made just below the lashes, and the skin is lifted and removed from the muscle to the rim of the bone. Fat and loose skin are taken out, and the incision is closed. The operation takes from sixty to ninety minutes and can be performed on an outpatient basis. The eyes remain covered for one or two hours—you are then free to leave. For the first thirty-six hours eyes must be sponged with ice water every ten minutes while you are awake, to control swelling and prevent bruising. After three days the stitches are taken out; after seven to ten days all signs of the operation are gone, and usual activities—including the use of eye makeup—can be resumed. There are virtually no visible scars, since all stitches are hidden in the normal folds of the skin.

Face lift

A full face lift—which smooths the lines from the nose to the corners of the mouth, tightens the lower half of the face, and firms the jowls—involves preoperative sedation, then local anesthesia. An incision is made, starting at the scalp above the ear, continuing down in the crease in front of the ear, curving up behind the earlobes and into the back of the scalp. Skin is cut loose from the underlying structures, lifted up, pulled tight, and the excess is removed before the incision is stitched closed. Operating time is about two hours—longer if ancillary surgery is included. The procedure can be performed on an outpatient basis or in

a hospital. After five days the ear stitches are taken out, after ten days scalp stitches are removed, and two or three weeks later, bruising and swelling are down. Scars are primarily hidden in the hairline, and there should be no visible pulling—tension is in the scalp. The stitches in front of the ear heal to a fine white line that can be covered by makeup.

Eye makeup—shadow, mascara, even false eyelashes—can be applied five days after the removal of the last stitches, foundation normally around the seventh day—with concealing cream to help mask any undereye bruises. Makeup removal should be gentle: best for eyes are oil-saturated pads, or oily cleanser on a cotton pad; for skin, tepid water and mild soap, thoroughly rinsed, followed by a moisturizer, because skin is very dry and in need of protection while healing.

Hair can be styled with a wide-toothed comb and warm water on the fourth day after surgery, but should not be shampooed until a week after surgery, with a very mild formulation in the shower or by an experienced expert. A hairdryer on a lukewarm setting should be used; rollers can be wound loosely. Hair coloring can be continued approximately three weeks after surgery.

Forehead lift

This operation is an extensive one—it reduces creases and furrows in the forehead, plus raises sagging eyebrows—and can be performed in conjunction with a face lift. Local anesthesia is commonly used, and surgery takes about one and a half hours. A slit is made behind the hairline, along the top of the scalp from ear to ear. Skin is pulled taut, a strip of the muscle is removed, and the incision is closed. Sutures are removed on the tenth day after surgery; there is no visible scarring.

Brow lift

This procedure corrects sagging brows but involves such extensive, visible scarring that many doctors do not perform it, preferring instead the forehead lift. A wedge of skin above the outer part of the eyebrows is removed and the brows raised so that the eyes are opened.

Chin lift

A double chin consisting of excess fatty tissue in the neck is removed via a small incision in a skin crease under the chin. This procedure can be done only in conjunction with a face lift and takes about twenty minutes to perform.

Platysma lift

Although the neck area is generally firmed and smoothed by a full face lift, sagging skin marked by vertical folds caused by displacement or stretching of the edge of the platysma, a superficial muscle of the neck, remains unchanged, so an additional operation is called for. Performed in conjunction with a face lift, the platysma lift involves splitting the muscle to the side or sides of the jaw and pulling the skin taut over it. It is a fairly recent development, and although initial results appear good, additional follow-up

time is needed before it becomes standard practice.

Elevating the nose tip

A drooping nose is one of the by-products of the maturing process. Raising the nose tip imperceptibly involves the cartilage only—the bone is not touched. This procedure often accompanies a face lift.

Shortening the earlobe

As we grow older our earlobes grow longer. Shortening them, by snipping off part of the skin, is an uncomplicated procedure that can be performed in conjunction with other surgery.

Zyderm collagen implants and fluid medical-grade silicone injections

These two substances are particularly effective for replacing lost tissue: plumping out deep lines in the forehead, crow's-feet, and other profound grooves where surgery would be either ineffective or too extensive. They are injected into the skin to bolster it from underneath, flattening scars and wrinkles. Zyderm is a new substance composed of a purified form of bovine (cow) collagen and considered by some doctors to still be experimental, since long-term results on its safety and efficacy (persistent benefits) will not be available for many years. However medical-grade silicone (dimethylpolysitoxane), explains Dr. Norman Orentreich, has been used for more than twenty-five years—safely. Problems have arisen when it was administered incorrectly and by unqualified, untrained people: it should never be directly injected into breast tissue, as it makes mammograms difficult to read and breast cancer more difficult to diagnose by palpation, and it must be absolutely pure without any additives. Some physicians treat with both fluid silicone and Zyderm; some prefer one over the other for different situations and different patients.

Zyderm is injected in gel form; it becomes fibrous, a part of the natural skin structure, forming a framework upon which skin can build. Since it is part water, there is swelling, but the skin falls back down. The number of treatments vary depending upon the severity of the wrinkling and the response of the individual. The literature indicates that allergic reaction to Zyderm is possible, and a test injection is required before treatment is begun.

Injections of micro-droplets of fluid medical-grade silicone replace lost tissues by stimulating your own skin cells to produce new collagen. Injections are administered at one- to six-month intervals in order to allow time for new collagen from previous injections to develop; silicone does not provoke an allergic reaction.

How long does plastic surgery last?

While in one sense the benefits of successful plastic surgery last a lifetime—you look better, younger than before—you can never stop the clock. The factors that caused you to consider surgery are always affecting your skin: the aging process, the pull of gravity, your emotions (happiness can make a lift last longer), life-style (alcohol causes puffy lids; rapid weight-loss taxes the skin), the sun (the fastest premature skin-ager), heredity. But how often you need surgery varies from one individual to another. Generally, though, the repeat cycle for a face lift is every eight years, but some surgeons believe that there is a limit to the benefits to be gained by successive operations. During a lift, stretch is removed from the skin and too much surgery, too much tightening, can result in a "mask" look—the loss of normal facial expression. This is something to keep in mind and discuss with your doctor.

A bit about body surgery

Age and the elements affect the skin of the body in the same manner as they do the face. The breasts, in particular, may sag and, since they contain no muscles, cannot be firmed by exercise. Abdominal skin, too, shows relaxation. Surgery can be performed, not to tone this area but rather to remove loose, hanging folds of skin caused by loss of weight or by pregnancy. Surgery for buttocks, thighs, upper arms, and hands is frowned upon by many experts, among them Dr. Herman, who cautions that severe scarring and the possibility of complications can be far worse than the conditions that would prompt you to consider surgery in the first place.

Abdominal surgery

Loose skin and the underlying muscles can be tightened, and stretch marks and scars below the navel can be removed by abdominal surgery, but the trade-off is substantial scarring. This surgery is performed under general anesthetic and takes about two to three hours. An incision is made across the lower abdomen and all of the skin below the navel is removed. The upper skin is brought down and stitched to close the incision. The navel remains intact and in position; a new opening is constructed for it. Although the scar around the navel generally fades, the lower abdominal scar is visible unless hidden by underwear or a bikini bottom.

Swelling of the lower abdominal skin and puffiness caused by accumulation of fluid beneath the skin disappear in approximately two weeks. Stitches are taken out seven to ten days after surgery, and the incision flattens several weeks later. Exercise can be resumed three weeks after surgery.

Breast lift

This three-hour operation to produce a more youthful shape is performed under general anesthesia. Breast skin is removed, and there is usually no change in nipple sensation or color. There will be scars around the areola (the pigmented area around the nipple), a scar from the areola down to the fold under the breast, and another in the fold under the breast—they fade to white lines in six to eight months. A specially designed brassiere has to be worn for about ten days, and exercise is prohibited for three weeks.

Breast reconstruction after mastectomy

Postmastectomy breast reconstruction usually involves insertion of a specially designed silicone implant to create the breast shape. This procedure takes about one and a half hours and is performed with a general anesthetic. Happily, almost all women who have had simple or modified radical mastectomies, and many who have had radicals, can benefit from it. The implant is inserted through an incision on the side of the chest under the arm. A halter-type bra is then worn continuously for ten days, until the stitches are removed. The nipple is reconstructed during the second stage of the operation, six weeks later after the normal blood supply returns to the chest skin. Most often, a portion of the opposite nipple and areola is used for reconstruction and gives the best cosmetic results. Stitches are removed after ten days, and you can exercise after two weeks. The implanted breast will be firmer and less mobile; it will approximate the opposite breast but cannot duplicate it. It does provide cleavage and looks natural even in a bathing suit. If fear of recurring cancer due to an implant is holding you back, be reassured that silicone implants have been used successfully for over thirty years without any evidence that they are cancer-causing. After a radical mastectomy, if the chest skin is extremely tight, your surgeon can transfer local tissue onto the chest prior to implant insertion. This procedure involves visible scarring and is less pleasing aesthetically. Dr.

Herman recommends that any woman considering a skin transfer should discuss it fully with her doctor, ask to see photographs of it, and give it extra thought.

How to find a plastic surgeon who is right for you

You cannot assess how these procedures will benefit you personally by reading about them. Plastic surgery may be a modern miracle, but it still involves irreversible changes in body tissue. And there are risks, made minimal in the hands of a skilled and trained surgeon, but you should be aware of them: bleeding, infection, scar overgrowth—even death. There is scarring; it may be hidden behind the hairline or virtually undetectable within the folds of the skin, or easily camouflaged with makeup. There is also pain and discomfort—although it is said to be surprisingly little. Your doctor should explain all of this at the initial consultation. But first you have to find the right doctor for you, one who is board certified or board eligible. Board certification indicates that the doctor received both basic and additional training and testing in plastic and reconstructive surgery and has passed a battery of tests to meet the standards set by the American Board of Plastic Surgery. "Board eligible" means completion of training and eligibility to take the examinations. Certification equals training; it does not, however, guarantee good results. Plastic surgery is an art as well as a science. The surgeon's skill, taste, sense of proportion, and artistic talent, combined with his schooling, make all the difference.

If you do not already know a reputable plastic surgeon, you can find one in the following ways:

—Consult the *Directory of Medical Specialists,* a two-volume set found in every library, which lists all board-certified plastic surgeons. Look under "Plastic Surgeons" or consult the alphabetical index at the end of Volume Two.

—Request a list of surgeons in your area from The American Society of Plastic and Reconstructive Surgeons at 29 East Madison Street, Suite 800, Chicago, Illinois 60602, (312) 641-0593, a professional organization to which the majority of certified plastic surgeons belong.

—Ask your family doctor or a friend satisfied with her surgery to recommend someone. Check the *Directory* for board certification.

—Call your local hospital or county medical society and request the names of board-certified or board-eligible doctors.

The initial consultation

At this point you may have several names, all board-certified, well affiliated, and, lucky you, highly recommended. How do you make a choice? "The initial consultation is extremely important," counsels Dr. Herman. "It's time for you to interview the doctor while he interviews you. You should feel that the doctor is concerned, is listening and cares about you. You should feel comfortable and like his attitude, his answers to your questions. Write your questions down so that you won't forget anything, and note the answers, too." You want to know his qualifications, whether the surgery under discussion is easy, reasonable, how long it takes and the changes you can expect, what the complications could be, the length of time you'll be bandaged, have stitches, whether the scars will be noticeable or extensive. If you are considering breast or abdominal surgery, ask to see photographs so you won't receive any postoperative rude shocks. "I am careful not to suggest additional surgery except when it is directly related to the operation under discussion and I can see that the patient may not realize the difference that, let's say, the slight elevation of her nose tip or chemical peeling above the lips might make during a face lift," continues Dr. Herman. "I would advise any woman to be wary of a doctor who advises entirely unrelated surgery—ears in addition to the nose, and the like." Now is the time to talk also about price and when you have to pay. Prices vary among doctors. Find out whether your medical insurance will cover any of your bills.

DERMATOLOGY

"Dryness and the development of small growths on the skin, little flat or raised brown spots, usually become noticeable after the age of forty, although they can happen earlier—but anyone over forty is susceptible. Wrinkling will be more prominent now as well. Especially after menopause, you'll notice changes in your skin. It may become drier and its texture will change," explains Dr. John Romano, attending dermatologist at the New York Hospital–Cornell Medical Center. Minor skin annoyances rather than the radical changes that would prompt surgery may warrant a visit to a dermatologist, who routinely treats growths, broken blood vessels, brown spots, scars and breakouts, and lines and wrinkles, as well as a variety of more serious problems including hair and scalp disorders and skin diseases. Many dermatologists, like plastic surgeons, perform dermabrasion and chemical peeling—procedures that were discussed in the preceding section—and inject Zyderm and fluid medical-grade silicone. Although their functions sometimes overlap, dermatologists often work closely with plastic surgeons. Your dematologist can probably, in fact, recommend a good plastic surgeon if you need one, and vice versa.

How a dermatologist can help your skin now, and later too

• *Lines and wrinkles*—"People with exaggerated facial expressions—those who frown or grimace frequently—may induce lining and wrinkling by simply stretching their skin. This is unavoidable. Genetic tendencies, aging, and wrinkling all move together as well. But the sun is the number one ager—I can't emphasize enough the need for people to minimize sun exposure," declares Dr. Romano, who suggests corrective surgery as the only means of treating severe wrinkling and considerable facial sagging. "For those bothered by minor to moderate wrinkling—between the nose and mouth, on the lower part of the cheek or around the eyes—and who do not want to undergo major plastic surgery, injection of bovine collagen is a feasible alternative," he offers. "It's not terribly painful, is much less expensive than surgery, and cures wrinkling as it occurs. It is not a solution for it, nor does it prevent further wrinkling." Fine lines also respond to dermabrasion and chemical peeling, most often around the lips, on the chin and cheeks, and lateral to the eyes.

• *Scars*—acne-scarred skin is often treated with dermabrasion or chemical peeling. Although skin color eventually evens out after a peeling, there is sometimes a line of dermarcation as a result of an increase in pigment. If it is marked, your doctor can prescribe a bleaching solution. Pinhole scars that are too deep to be corrected by peeling are often filled in with a plug of skin taken from behind the ear, then abraded to blend in with the skin around them.

• *Brown spots*—these small, slightly raised dark spots are concentrations of pigment cells, topped by an overgrowth of skin cells. "They are a normal occurrence—genetically caused—although sometimes induced by the sun," explains Dr. Romano. "Everyone is going to get a few, but when you get a lot, even though you have not been out in the sun, they tend to be genetic. If they are continually irritated, they should be removed." Flat brown spots can often be bleached with a solution prescribed by your dermatologist, as it contains a higher percentage of hydroquinone, the bleaching agent, than an over-the-counter preparation. Raised spots can be burned off by electrosurgery—an electric current passes through a needle, causing a spark to jump between the tip and the skin, burning it. A scab forms, and when it falls off, the skin underneath is clear. Raised spots can also be frozen with liquid nitrogen so that they peel off. When there is an abundance of them on the face, a light chemical peeling or dermabrasion yields good results.

• *Red lines*—these tiny lines around the nose and cheeks are caused by blood flowing through dilated blood vessels. They can be sealed off by electrosurgery, which is very effective. Although the tendency toward them is inherited, they can be brought about by factors that cause the blood vessels to expand: by alcohol, coffee, tea, and cola because they contain vasodilators, as well as by very hot or spicy foods, constant exposure to extreme warmth (including sunbathing), high blood pressure, a blow to the skin, and hormonal changes during menopause.

For professional cleansing and

care many dermatologists now employ aestheticians in their offices; others routinely advise facials with a qualified specialist and emphasize their therapeutic and psychological benefits. "After all," cites one, "pampering can relieve stress, and whatever makes you feel good can make your skin look better."

The salon facial

"A professional facial is a necessary part of a good skin-care program," says Lydia Sarfati of the Klisar Skin Care Center. "It's like brushing your teeth—to keep them healthy you have to do it at home on a regular basis, but you still need a professional cleaning every few months." A professional skin cleansing removes the surface debris that builds up faster after forty, which clogs the pores and clouds the complexion, making it look tired and prematurely old.

What can you expect from a good facial? "It should be a relaxing and pleasant experience," Lydia says. And should always start with an analysis to determine your skin type. "If it doesn't, I suggest you get up and leave, because you won't get what your individual skin needs—you'll be just a number. Analysis defines the treatment that follows."

Although every complexion differs, the steps after analysis usually include:
• Massage to relax the shoulders, neck, and facial muscles—it should be very gentle, light; there should be no tugging, pulling, or discomfort.
• Cleansing, which involves steaming the skin to open the pores, then removal of blackheads and whiteheads.
• A light "peeling" with an abrasive cream or mask to lift off dead cells—the slowdown in cell turnover after forty results in a dulling surface layer. Its buildup can be prevented by exfoliation so that the skin looks more radiant.
• Masks, to hydrate and balance the moisture level of the skin.

The entire procedure takes between one and one and a half hours, and your skin should look refreshed, clearer and smoother. On Lydia's avoidance list for skin at this age are: vigorous massage and peel-off masks, which stretch and pull the skin, encouraging broken capillaries; extremes of hot and cold following each other, which unduly shock the system; and treatment with an electric current, which can be especially irritating if skin is sensitive.

She suggests the following pointers for deciding if a salon can give you the results you want:
• Before making an appointment, ask for a complimentary consultation—most salons offer them.
• Look over the facilities. Check if they are clean, pleasing. You want a quiet, restful environment.
• Meet the person who is administering the facial. You should feel comfortable with her.
• Check credentials—where she has studied, her years of experience.
• Ask about the products used and what they contain. This is very helpful if you have allergies. Avoid products that are perfumed: they are irritating.

• Look for a salon that leans toward a holistic approach—the mind-body connection is very important.

• Remember that a facial should never hurt. There may be a little discomfort if you are having blackheads extracted, but there should never be pain, bruising, or bleeding. And price is no indication of service.

"But no specialist is a magician," Lydia adds. "A facial once a month does not grant you carte blanche to ignore your skin. You have to maintain it yourself, every day at home: cleanse it, tone and moisturize it, exfoliate it when necessary. You must take precautions in the sun, drink a lot of water, eat correctly, and exercise. Skin health and overall health go together—and having a positive attitude about yourself is vital!"

Acupuncture rejuvenation

"I classify cosmetic acupuncture somewhere between a facial and a face lift," explains Dr. Adam Lewenberg, who practices internal medicine and acupuncture in New York City. "With it, I can temporarily reverse to some degree the aging process of the subcutaneous tissue; I can lessen lines and wrinkles, improving the quality of the skin by stimulating and increasing the blood supply and circulation in the facial area, and by tightening most of the facial muscles. I can also alleviate tension and depression, which are, in most cases, the underlying causes of facial wrinkles." He uses acupuncture to treat the whole person, stating that a youthful look involves more than a line-free face—it encompasses walk, movements, the ability to relax, and lack of pain from illness. "Acupuncture can relieve pain, restore normal activity, and help a woman to help herself feel rejuvenated, look rejuvenated."

This four-thousand-year-old Chinese practice of inserting special needles at nerve-impulse points on the body to lessen pain and certain problems connected with aging, Dr. Lewenberg is quick to add, cannot replace the surgical face lift. "Acupuncture can be used by a woman to delay aging if she can't afford or doesn't want surgery. It can also be helpful before or after an operation as an adjunct to it, because it improves the quality of the skin, which surgery cannot do." To what extent it acts on lines depends on skin type, though—obviously some faces are more sensitive than others. But even if it cannot smooth wrinkles, it can promote a better, younger overall look.

In what mysterious ways acupuncture works, not even the experts know exactly. It is believed to release the body's own pain-killing secretions and also to activate the brain areas regulating the emotions, to ease stress and anxiety and all kinds of nervous mannerisms. Dr. Lewenberg administers acupuncture to suppress certain cravings—for food, drugs, alcohol, and smoking. Smoking, he states, is particularly insidious, as nicotine decreases circulation to the subcutaneous tissues and causes changes in the small blood vessels, increasing the aging of the skin. "Tension and smoking seem to go together—how much of wrinkling is due to smoking and how much to stress is hard to say. We know that if we can control both tension and smoking, we can improve a woman's looks.

"In order for rejuvenation through acupuncture to be successful, though," he emphasizes, "it has to be combined with all the other factors I have discussed—a healthy lifestyle, including exercise and diet, emotional tranquillity, freedom from pain, and avoidance of harmful habits like smoking."

COSMETIC DENTISTRY

"Cosmetic dentistry can smooth wrinkles on the cheeks and around the mouth when they are the result of missing or malpositioned teeth," says Dr. Gary Soldati, a leading New York cosmetic dentist, who often works hand in hand with plastic surgeons. "We insert a bridge or a denture that's slightly built out—we call it 'plumping'—it fills in the concave cheek area and gives a beautiful architecture to the face. Molars in the back of the mouth can also be built out, but carefully, or the jaw will look boxy."

The cosmetic dentist is another one of the medical wizards who can help your face—by helping your teeth—look better forever. "If you take care of your teeth properly, they should last a lifetime," stresses Dr. Soldati. "Full dentures, thank goodness, are getting to be a thing of the past. People who care about their teeth, care for them, and usually never need dentures." Teeth do, however, appear to yellow slightly

with age. An improper brushing technique coupled with too abrasive a toothpaste can thin the enamel, letting dentin—a yellowish tissue that forms the body of the tooth—show through. More commonly, though, it causes gum recession showing exposed dentin. At the same time, the enamel, as it is ever so slightly porous, is stained by food and drink: blueberries, red wine, all artificial coloring—and nicotine. But yellowing is not really the problem; missing teeth, cracked, rotated, or unaesthetically contoured teeth, or those shortened due to grinding, are, and cosmetic dentistry can solve all of them:

• Crowning: This method involves first filing the tooth, then fitting it with a jacket or crown, usually in porcelain. If teeth are missing, a bridge can be made and cemented to the adjacent teeth, which are capped to hold it permanently in place. But artistry must be combined with technical expertise, in the front of the mouth especially. "What you want to avoid are teeth that look like a row of piano keys," says Dr. Soldati. "Teeth should not be white, nor perfect—they have to have the slightest colorations or imperceptible rotations, imperfections. The dentist has to imitate the impression of nature, something believable, otherwise they will look fake. The center of the tooth should be slightly lighter than the root, the tiny mutations, the translucent blue around its edges all have to be very subtle. And it has to go under the gumline just so." A crowned tooth should match the teeth on either side of it; in the case of a full set of crowns, teeth can be two shades lighter if they work with hair and skin tone.

• Implants: There are several types of implants, but basically the procedure involves securing a metal material with a protrusion post inside or over the bones of the jaw. The post is then crowned and can be connected to the remaining teeth. In the near future, implants may be in all cases useful replacements for removable dentures, if there are no natural teeth to support an appliance. Today, however, they are not always successful. They are often rejected by the bone and loosen.

• Bonding: This relatively new procedure involves laying a veneer over the teeth to mask discolorations, chips, breaks, splits, and spaces. The enamel is first etched with acid so that it is porous. After that, a claylike tooth-colored dental material is laid on, which is hardened and bonded to the tooth by ultraviolet or white light. It is then carved and polished. Advantages are that the tooth underneath does not have to be cut down, making bonding a good solution when the problem is a minor one. Should all of the teeth need covering, Dr. Soldati comments, "Bonding is wonderful in many cases, but the ultimate cosmetic result, I am sorry to say, falls short of crowning with porcelain. Since the bonding substance is acrylic-like and porous, I find that it picks up stains and discolorations and has to be re-done every few years to look best. It also becomes opaque—sacrificing a most essential translucency." Bonding seems to hold great promise for the future, however, and with time and research may eventually be perfected for all cases.

When lines around the corners of the mouth are the result of an incorrect bite, orthodontia—moving the teeth—may be the answer, because once the bite is adjusted, so are the lines. There are a variety of techniques that alter the position of the teeth—several are invisible, removal, or both. An orthodontist is the specialist you should consult.

Caring for your teeth

"Any alteration of the teeth affects the periodontal relationship," explains Dr. David L. Hoexter, New York periodontist and chief of periodontia at the Hospital for Joint Diseases. "The more dentistry you have done in your mouth, the more you're changing nature, interrupting its balance. Compensation by way of thorough and proper oral hygiene is essential."

The number one dental problem at this stage of life—and the greatest cause of tooth loss—is periodontal disease, which infects the tissue around the tooth, then breaks down the bone structure. "Periodontal disease is not hereditary; it's caused by improper mouth hygiene," continued Dr. Hoexter, "which allows the buildup of plaque—a mixture of saliva and bacteria—between and around the teeth. After one day, the plaque calcifies and can't be removed by anyone except a trained expert." That is why it's imperative for you to clean your teeth thoroughly at least once a day, preferably at night—but two times daily is even better. Although periodontal disease is usually accompanied by bad breath, spacing between the front teeth, and bleeding and swollen gums, the latter two may not be evident. "The gingeva [the medical term for gums] does not always give clear warning of the disease, so it is important to have your dentist probe it during each checkup," Dr. Hoexter advises.

"Proper oral hygiene means rubbing the teeth," he says. "This is the only way to break up the bacterial plaque." Rubbing should involve a combination of brushing and flossing, since normal brushing usually misses most of the plaque. One day, check your mouth with a disclosing tablet after you've brushed to see exactly how ineffective it is, unless preceded by flossing. You might want to use a perio aid as well, to get between the teeth.

• Dental floss: should be the first step—vital for cleaning between the teeth and under the gums, places a toothbrush cannot reach. Unwaxed floss is best, wrapped around the tooth to gently rub off film. Use a floss threader to get under bridgework and around teeth that are positioned very close together.

• Your toothbrush: should have soft nylon bristles that are rounded at the tips. A child's size may be best to work into all spaces and around gums. Angle bristles toward the gum and move them gently back and forth at the gumline, reaching under it. Replace your toothbrush frequently.

• Dental irrigators: do not remove plaque but can be helpful in flushing out food particles between the teeth and under any bridgework, after flossing and brushing.

Supplement at-home care with frequent professional cleanings and checkups—always have your dentist probe for gum disease. Watch your diet, too—try to avoid sugar and white flour, foods that encourage the formation of plaque. Concentrate instead on do-gooders like apples, celery, and carrots, which clean as well as strengthen the teeth.

Chapter 7

Controlling the Skin-aging Factors

She looks fifty; you look thirty-five. Yet you're both forty. What are you doing right? What is she doing wrong? How can you keep your skin looking younger than you are? Facial aging is related to certain external factors, which is why skin does not mature at a predetermined rate like the internal organs—the lungs, heart, liver. "Sun exposure plays a big part in skin aging," says Dr. John Romano. "I can't say that at a certain year the skin will look a certain way. If you took a biopsy from the buttock of both a sixty-year-old woman and a thirty-year-old, you would probably not be able to tell the difference between them."

If you look at your mother's face, you can get some idea of how yours will appear at her age—provided you treat it in the same manner she did. What you do to your skin can hasten premature aging—or slow it down. Although your pattern of wrinkling is genetically programmed at birth along with bone structure and coloring, the way you live will determine the depth of these wrinkles, thus their visibility later on in life. And thanks to a new and improved understanding of how skin functions and ages, many of the changes that were once considered inevitable can be put off for years, perhaps even forever.

THE FACTORS THAT AFFECT YOUR SKIN'S AGE AND HOW TO OFFSET THEM

Sun exposure

"How can something that makes me look so good, be so bad for me?" you ask. For it's true that a tan can be attractive—it masks skin imperfections, gives a healthy glow, and at first flush the slight swelling that follows exposure smoothes out facial lines. But the trade-off for this "healthy" bronze hue can be wrinkles, sagging, broken blood vessels, dryness, and blotchiness—all symptoms usually associated with aging. Now, through medical research, we know that these signs are the result of chronic sun damage rather than some inevitable deterioration. The sun ages skin faster than time does. And it ages skin after forty faster than it does skin at twenty. When exposed to the sun, your skin thickens. It tries to protect itself by building a barrier layer of cells. At the same time, for added protection, pigment cells produce more melanin (pigment). But your skin becomes more sun-sensitive as the years go by, it gets sheerer, and with each passing decade there is a 10 to 20 percent decrease in pigment cells, so your natural protection wears thin.

Ultraviolet rays promote more than tanned, thickened skin, they penetrate deep into the skin's layers to frazzle the collagen fibers. When you were twenty, damaged collagen could be absorbed while new collagen was continually forming, but now collagen production has slowed down. These broken fibers cause the skin to lose flexibility, it sags and wrinkles. And that's not all. The chemical reaction produced by ultraviolet rays can result in improperly formed cells, giving rise to benign growths and, sometimes, malignant ones—skin cancer rarely appears on those parts of the body shielded from the sun. And there is now some indication that these rays also damage the body's immune system, its natural mechanism of self-defense against disease. Findings show that even a mild sunburn changes vital elements of the system that are present in circulating blood. Certain conditions could then be activated that the immune system would not be able to reject, as in the case of cancers.

Skin dries out from the sun's heat—it coarsens, flakes, and mottles, making lines and wrinkles appear deeper. Moisturizers can ease but can't treat this dehydration, since they only seal in water, they don't replace it.

All of the above are valid reasons why a sunscreen should be your single most important beauty and health aid, in summer or whenever you are facing the sun. You'll find sunscreens in sun preparations and in cosmetics, too—moisturizers, foundations, lipsticks, blushers and eye shadows—as companies realize that the future of youthful-looking skin lies in ultraviolet protection.

The sun preparation you choose, however, should have a high sun protection factor (SPF), preferably a 10 to 15. This numerical rating indicates the degree of protection the product offers—the higher the number, the more the protection. With a 10, for example, you can stay in the sun ten times longer without burning than you could if you wore no protection. Thus, if you normally redden after fifteen minutes, with an SPF 10 you can stay in the sun a hundred and forty minutes with the same result. Every skin, even if dark, even if already tanned, needs protection. Despite all the warnings, if you feel that a blush of tan gives you a psychological advantage, take these necessary precautions in the sun:

• Tan slowly so that your skin can protect itself; color will last longer. Begin with a higher SPF, then change numbers as your skin acquires a base tan.

• Consider latitude: the nearer you live to the sun, the shorter the amount of time it takes to burn. Consider altitude, too: the higher you are, the less atmosphere there is to filter out ultraviolet rays, so you burn faster. Always use a sunscreen.

• You are less likely to burn early in the morning and late in the afternoon, when the sun's strength is weakest. The most damaging hours are from eleven to two.

• Limit sunbathing to no longer

than two hours at a time, even if you are already tan and wearing protection. The sun's heat is very dehydrating.

• Ultraviolet rays cut through fog and clouds; you can burn when the day is overcast.

• You need sunscreen protection even when you're covered up—the sun penetrates a thin T-shirt, for example, wet or dry. Sand reflects rays even if you are under an umbrella, while water conducts them—so you need a formulation with staying power.

• Water and perspiration reduce a sunscreen's effectiveness—reapply frequently, particularly after swimming.

• Never use a sun reflector.

• Antibiotics, some barbiturates, oil of bergamot (found in perfume), and certain foods like limes, carrots, and celery, can make skin more susceptible to burning.

• Avoid burning by playing a sport—a moving target is harder for rays to single out than an immobile one.

• Cheat on your tan. Protect your face with a sun-block but tan your body lightly, then use a facial bronzing gel so the two will match.

• Follow your sunbath with a lavish smoothing of moisturizer over damp skin to offset drying.

Rapid weight loss

Losing a lot of weight quickly is the second most serious skin ager. Your skin is not elastic enough to snap back into shape, as it might have twenty years ago, so it sags and folds. If you want to slim down, diet—but drop pounds slowly. Your skin can then make the adjustment and shrink accordingly. And weight lost this way usually stays off, your ultimate goal! More about dieting—plus a plan that will help you keep your looks while losing weight—in Chapter 11.

How you eat also shows on your skin; a big change in your diet will be reflected in skin tone and texture. Stick to a plan rich in complex carbohydrates, with adequate amounts of protein and balanced portions of dairy products and grains. Steer clear of refined and processed foods—they tend to be high in calories and salt and low in vitamins. Cut down on caffeine because it depletes vitamins and minerals from your body.

Be sure to include adequate portions of the foods listed below, as they contain vitamins and minerals needed by your skin to stay glowing and healthy. The subject of supplemental vitamins is an unresolved one. Reportedly there is no conclusive evidence that they will improve your skin, but vitamin deficiencies will certainly be noticeable. Best—eat a well-rounded and nutritionally balanced diet.

• Vitamin A: aids in preventing scaling, itching, and dryness. Found in yellow fruits and vegetables—carrots, sweet potatoes, peaches; dark leafy vegetables—spinach and parsley; calf's liver. *Note:* Vitamin A tablets can be toxic when taken in large doses.

• Vitamin B: important for smooth skin; deficiencies can result in dryness and flakiness. Found in brewer's yeast, brown rice, bananas, lean meat, green vegetables, whole grain cereals and breads.

• Vitamin C: the collagen builder, necessary for keeping skin elastic and supple. Found in citrus fruits, broccoli, kale, cabbage, and parsley.

• Iron: needed for healthy color and prevention of anemia, which makes skin pale and dry. Found in liver, shellfish, nuts, egg yolks.

• Vitamin E: believed to improve skin tone by working against the breakdown of inner cell structures. Found in safflower, wheat germ, and corn oils.

Water should be a basic of any diet—it's an element essential for maintaining the hydration of the system, the skin. It flushes out toxins and keeps the complexion from dehydrating. Try to drink between six and eight glasses daily.

The environment

Dried-out skin feels rough, looks prematurely old. Your complexion needs moisture to stay soft and supple, but extremes of weather—variations in temperature and humidity—can deplete its natural moisture. In winter this problem is particularly severe because low temperatures accompanied by low humidity and wind cut down on skin's elasticity and speed up moisture loss. Moving between dry, overheated air indoors and windy, freezing air outdoors will quickly parch skin more, especially if it is unprotected. Moisturizing is very important now—for both comfort and appearance. Explains Dr. Romano, "Rubbing dry or itchy skin will exaggerate wrinkling and cause coarseness—you want to keep it moisturized and comfortable." In summer the drying combination of the sun's heat and air conditioning makes moisturizing a must. And the older you get, the more moisturizing you need, because moisture retention ability and oil gland function (oil is the skin's natural moisture-sealer) decline with age, making you more susceptible to moisture loss.

Important, too, is adding more moisture to the environment. Turn the thermostat down in winter; in summer, keep air conditioning to a minimum. Surround yourself with moisture-loving greenery and invest in a humidifier. "If I were to cite the single best skin investment you could make, it would be a cold-steam vaporizer placed in the room where you sleep," says one leading doctor. "It adds the humidity needed to keep skin healthy and leaves no sickroom odor like hot steam."

Keep skin from wrinkling by helping it to retain water from the inside—drink lots of fluids to replace those lost through evaporation, respiration, and perspiration. Apply moisturizer over damp skin—and when flying, since the compressed air in planes is particularly dehydrating, refresh and rehydrate your face by misting it frequently with mineral water.

Along with sunlight and the weather, pollution is the third environmental enemy. Dirt and chemicals in the air accumulate on the skin's surface, clouding and irritating it. In fact, the long-term effects of some of these chemicals are not even yet known—but you can protect against them by cleansing properly and placing a protective barrier on your skin's surface—a moisturizer or sunscreen or both.

Smoking

If you haven't already stopped smoking for your health, you should for your skin—cigarettes add years to your looks by encouraging lines, wrinkles, and sallowness.

Skin's healthy pink hue is due in part to the blood circulating just beneath its surface, blood that brings it food and oxygen to keep cells vital; blood that carries away the wastes that clog and cloud the complexion. Smoking inhibits this essential circulation, impeding the oxygenation of the cells, thus affecting skin's color and tone, contributing to lines and wrinkles. The continual mechanical action of pursing the lips to grip a cigarette and squinting the eyes to avoid smoke also leads to lines and wrinkles in both these areas.

Alcohol

Alcohol dehydrates the system, drawing water out of the tissues where it is needed to keep skin soft, smooth, and springy. At the same time, it interferes with the absorption of vitamins, so that the complexion becomes poorly nourished, losing vitality. Alcohol also constricts the blood flow, aggravating any predisposition toward broken blood vessels. And because it is initially a stimulant, although ultimately a depressant, it may interfere with sleep—a factor essential for a radiant, healthy look.

Limit your alcohol intake to no more than ten glasses (or fifteen ounces) weekly, and whenever you imbibe, try to counteract alcohol's dehydrating effects by drinking large amounts of water.

Stress

How many of your lines are the result of stress? Perhaps many more than you think. Stress stimulates the nerves to contract the muscles—a clenched jaw, pursed lips, furrowed brow—and the skin above them wrinkles. (Perhaps that's why everyone looks younger and more refreshed after a problem-free vacation.) If these muscle contractions continue over a long period of time, the wrinkles become permanent.

Your skin reflects your inner health, and stress can throw the system off-balance. In fact, with few exceptions stress and your reaction to it are considered the main cause of illness—skin disorders included. Stress can alter the hormone balance and since hormones regulate the look of skin—its color, tone, firmness, temperature, circulation, oil gland activity, new cell production, and hair growth—the results can include breakouts, mottling, oiliness, dryness or flakiness—the list goes on. Stress can further upset skin by disturbing the immune system, which controls susceptibility to infection and allergic reactions. While a certain amount of stress is healthy, necessary for coping with daily life, and unavoidable for solving problems (i.e. "creative anxiety"), it often has to be reduced to a more manageable level. Thus, learning how to relax is paramount to your health and your looks.

Sports and vigorous physical exercise distribute stress evenly; they serve as outlets for mounting tension and pent-up emotion. Although you may feel lethargic under stress, your muscles really want to move—give them a workout and they will relax, thus reducing anxiety. Seeing a movie, changing your environment, even daydreaming are also effective stress-relievers. Professional facials and body massages are especially soothing, as well as relaxation techniques like the following:

• *Deep breathing*—stand comfortably, then take a deep breath and hold it for 5 seconds. Exhale slowly, telling all your muscles to relax. You can do this anywhere—at any time, for a stress-free pause.

• *Mental relaxation*—lie down or stand or sit comfortably with your eyes closed. Let ideas float through your mind. Say no to them—and picture a calm blue sky or sea. Become aware of your slow, natural breathing. Think of a simple or comforting word or syllable. Keep the muscles around your eyes and forehead and mouth loose. Concentrate on keeping your forehead cool.

• *Shoulder rolls*—shrug the shoulders high, bringing them as close to your ears as you can. Roll them back, bring them forward, then straight up again. Repeat full circles four times, then reverse direction.

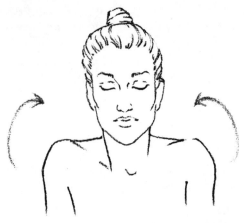

• *Meditation*—this technique popular in transcendental meditation allows your body to enter a deep state of rest. It can be practiced anywhere, but you might want to begin in a quiet, secluded spot. Choose a meaningless sound to concentrate on, like *om* or *shom*. Sit in a chair with your back straight and your head erect, keeping your hands loose in your lap; take several deep breaths. Close your eyes and repeat the sound, concentrating on it so that no other thoughts can enter your mind. Continue for 5 minutes. When you are finished, open your eyes, take a deep breath, and stretch.

• *Muscle relaxation*—lie in bed, keeping the room dark, with your head raised slightly on a pillow. Keep your arms close to the body, with your palms up. Keep eyes closed. Legs—begin with your left leg, then right:

• bend your foot forward, pointing toes without lifting the foot. Hold for a minute, then let go. Your foot will relax automatically.

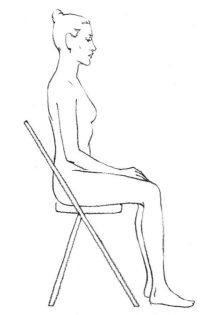

• bend your foot back toward your knee, keeping heels flat. Hold. Relax.

• straighten your leg as much as you can and tighten your thigh. Hold. Relax.

• bend your knee and bring your calf to your thigh. Hold. Relax. Change legs and repeat the series.

Torso

• pull in your abdomen and feel your torso contract. Hold for a minute, then relax.

• arch your spine. Hold. Relax.

• breathe in deeply and hold for several seconds before letting go of the breath with a deep sigh. Relax.

Arms—first left, then right.

• bend your hand back, palms are up. Hold. Relax.

• bend your hand forward. Hold. Relax.

• tense your entire arm as tightly as you can without moving it. Hold. Relax slowly until your arm is totally relaxed. Change arms and repeat the series.

Neck

• tilt your head slowly to the left, then the right, then forward, then back.

Forehead

• frown as hard as you can. Hold. Relax your forehead.

Hormonal activity

Widespread hormonal changes—most notably estrogen loss—that accompany menopause can result in a number of visible differences. Skin may become thinner and less firm; its texture coarser, drier, scalier. While hair on the head may fall out, facial hair can grow. Hormonal supplements—Estrogen Replacement Therapy—to reverse the effects of menopause are a solution some women and their physicians have turned to. But there is still much controversy about this treatment, with many experts believing that the risks of taking estrogens outweigh any benefits for all but a few post-menopausal women. Side effects of this therapy, however, are improved skin tone and texture and a halt to facial hair growth—but they are certainly not reasons enough to request or receive it.

Moisturizing helps to relieve dryness and scaliness, while excess facial hair responds to electrolysis,

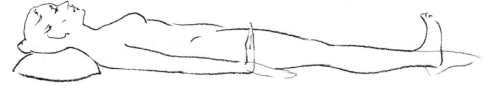

tweezing, and bleaching. Waxing and chemical depilatories are ideal on body skin but not recommended for the face—waxing pulls the skin and depilatories are too harsh and irritating.

• *Electrolysis*—This is the only method that removes hair permanently. It is effective for coarse hair in small areas. It is important to select a skilled expert, because improperly performed electrolysis can scar. A fine needle, through which an electric current passes, is inserted into the hair follicle to destroy the root. The new insulated bulbous probe is considered safest—its rounded end pierces the follicle but not the skin. This method is painful, but to what degree depends upon the sensitivity of your skin. Repeated sessions are necessary to destroy the hair root completely. The treated hair never grows back, but it always is possible that new growth can begin in an area that has undergone electrolysis.

• *Tweezing*—tweezing efficiently removes stray hairs anywhere on the face, provided there are not a lot of them. Regrowth can take up to three months, because the hair is pulled out below the hairline. Before and after tweezing, the area around the hairs should be cleansed with alcohol to lessen the risk of inflammation.

• *Bleaching*—if facial hair is fine, bleaching can lighten it, making it less noticeable. A facial hair preparation should be used, preceded by a patch test to determine allergic reaction. Bleaching lasts from four to six weeks.

Hormone creams are rarely prescribed for the face since the estrogen they contain can be absorbed into the skin, with results that may be potentially harmful. These creams cause the tissues to expand, plumping the skin so it feels smoother and softer. The same benefits, however, can be achieved with a rich emollient moisturizer, especially when it is applied over damp skin.

Exercise

The better you feel, the better you'll look. Exercise is one of the most positive factors in countering the aging process of the skin and other organs. It works the heart, stimulates the blood flow, boosts deep breathing—and this means increased nutrients, oxygen, and moisture to the skin. Sweating from exercise allows the skin to expel oils, salts, and water with increased efficiency, thus cleansing itself.

If you have not exercised before, start slowly and increase your time and effort very gradually. (More about exercise in Chapter 12.) Sports like swimming, fast walking, and jogging can be continued throughout a lifetime with positive results at every age. Proponents of jogging, in fact, believe that it inhibits wrinkles because it helps to control weight fluctuations that contribute to sagging skin.

While body exercise is indispensable for the face, facial exercises are believed by experts to be a waste of time. They may even do more harm than good. "Exercising the muscles causes the skin to stretch," explains Dr. Steven Herman, "increasing the possibility of lines and wrinkles."

Sleep

If you've ever fought off sleep, you know what a physical strain it is—and how aging it looks. Your facial muscles tense so that lines deepen; color drains from the face—the result of a chemical response in the body that can cause a lack of adequate blood flow to the skin. Sleep is indispensable for your total well-being, your face included. And how you sleep is more important than how much.

Sleeping on your face can etch in lines and wrinkles. Sleeping with your head flat can cause facial swelling and puffing, around the eyes especially. Best is sleeping on your back with the head of the bed elevated a few inches to keep body fluids from flowing back toward the face so that it swells. The quality of sleep counts too. Think back over the times you've awakened exhausted, even after seven hours of sleep. Looking and feeling refreshed in the morning occurs only when you've fallen asleep relaxed and have slept soundly for several hours. If you have difficulty sleeping, one or more of these methods might help:

• Exercise—you have to be fatigued enough muscularly to enjoy a good night's sleep. But a workout in the evening, for the purpose of sleeping well, should not be too strenuous or it will keep you awake.
• Avoid stimulants at night—no caffeine or alcohol or stimulating mental activity, which can also keep you awake.
• Try to maintain a fixed retiring and arising schedule.

• In bed, relax by taking your mind off problems and concentrating on happy thoughts. Unwind in a warm bath, indulge in a few of the relaxation methods discussed earlier in this chapter.
• Relieve an occasional bad night by taking two aspirin.
• Drink a glass of warm milk—it contains an essential amino acid called L-tryptophan, which has sedative powers. It's also found in meat and fish.
• Don't panic if you can't sleep. Watch television or read a good book. A night here and there without sleep will not damage your health—or looks. When your system really needs sleep, you will be able to sleep.
• See a qualified hypnotherapist about sleep self-hypnosis techniques if you have recurring sleep problems.
• Sleeping pills should be a last resort—they do not change sleep habits. Their chronic use can actually cause sleep problems. Do not repeatedly take any sleep aid—even an over-the-counter one—without first discussing its effects with your doctor.

Medication

Certain medicines change skin color and texture—ask your doctor what to expect from anything prescribed. Antibiotics, for example, can bring about a photosensitive reaction—you can develop a rash in the sun—while other medications are known to cause facial hair growth, hair fallout, itching, and additional discomforts that keep skin from looking its best.

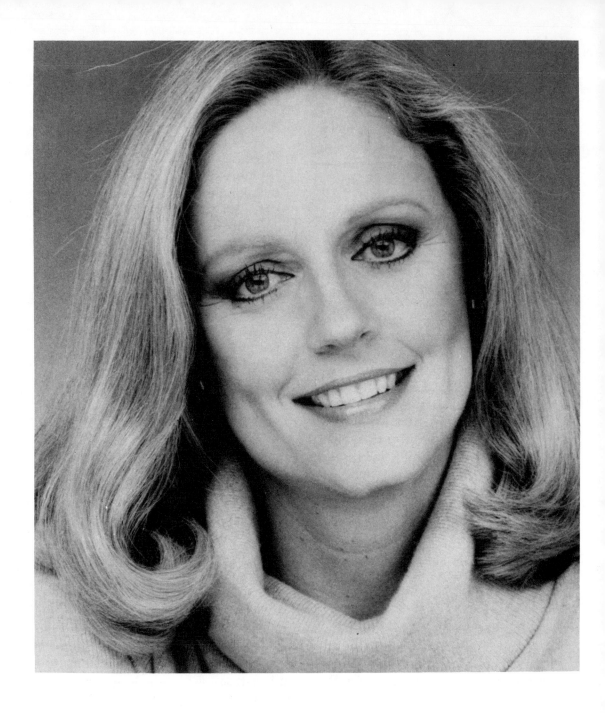

Sunny Griffin

Actress and television personality

I think I look forty. I have lines around my eyes, but I worked for them! The public image of what forty is, is wrong. There's a cultural lag. Forty means vital, healthy, and young. Forty looks fabulous. Things really get going at forty. Women improve with age, there's no doubt. I can't imagine why anyone was interested in me at eighteen. I wouldn't have been. I know who I am now. I know my limits; I'm confident and have the courage to try things. I'm not afraid of the unknown. I've taken chances and failed—and lived through the failures.

When I was in my twenties, I had no idea who I was. At that time I only wanted fame. Even when I was the highest-paid model in the world in 1966, I was groping for an identity. In my thirties I had achieved enough fame. I wanted to make a good living. I had a child and a bad marriage. Actually, I was divorced in my twenties, remarried and divorced again in my thirties, then married again—to my first husband. At age thirty-five I took a job as an executive—fashion and beauty director of Avon. But then, five years later, approaching forty, I wanted to get out. I knew who I was and I was miserable in my job. I wanted to go into show business. I had always wanted to be an actress.

It's funny, but even when I was so successful as a model, I never thought of myself as beautiful. I simply photographed well. I was the ugly girl in the world of beautiful girls. I was advised to have my nose fixed, but I'm glad I didn't. Strong bones keep you looking young. My imperfections began getting more interesting with age, while all those beautiful perfect girls were getting less beautiful. I'd say we were about even in looks at thirty.

I'm going to be the best at sixty. A lot of that confidence comes from being comfortable in my own body. I don't hate myself. If there's something I don't like, I do something about it. For example, I work hard at staying fit. I want to challenge my body, but that has to do in large part with the frustration that my body can do less. My flexibility is not what it used to be. In spite of these changes I'm in better shape now than I was in my twenties. But I work out more now. In my twenties I exercised only two or three times a week. Now it's six or more times. Plus I work harder. It's easier to stay fit than to become fit, but I feel that I'll be able to exercise even in my eighties.

When I had my two children—one at thirty-two, the other at thirty-five—I got very fat. I had to get my body back together—it took four years the last time. I'm an exercise nut. Tennis, skiing. For years I went to a gym, but today, dance is the answer. I had always been interested in dance, but I didn't start taking daily classes until I was thirty-eight. I used to worry about my inner thighs when I was very young; well, I don't have to these days. My legs are tight, my muscles are long and lean. I weigh 126 pounds, but I look thinner than I did at 122, because of all my muscle. My body is hard as a rock.

I think you should do whatever exercise turns you on. If you like to run, run. If you have to force yourself to work out, maybe you need music. But you should listen to your body; you don't want to damage it.

I watch what I eat. I haven't had red meat in years. Animal protein is important for building bulk, but I feel I have enough bulk. My diet is high in carbohydrates. I have boundless energy. I love fresh fruit and vegetables, and a lot of seafood. I drink wine, but I don't smoke.

As I get older, I find I can look younger with no makeup. When you have lines, powder is aging, but I need it for television. I look younger on television than I do in sharp still pictures. My hair is a little blonder now for TV. I haven't noticed any changes in my skin. It's never been wonderful. I used to baby it, but now I scrub with soap and a Buf-Puf and my skin looks better. I use lots of moisturizer—Clinique Subskin Creme. I still get pimples. I like to say that I went directly from pimples to wrinkles without a second in between, and an awful lot of overlap. I also like the sun, but I know how to tan. I'm naturally very yellow—one hour is enough to get me dark. I don't roast and I never wear clothes when I'm sunbathing. Since there are very few places one can sunbathe naked, I'm not in the sun very much. I change my makeup seasonally as my skin color changes.

I believe absolutely in plastic surgery. I had both my upper and lower eyelids done—droopy lids and early bagging is hereditary in my family—when I was seven months pregnant. Just ten days later I was photographed for a magazine cover. I felt like I had a new lease on life. I would have a face lift. I work hard at taking care of my body—and hate the idea of a young body but not a young face. I don't want to look younger, but just as good as I can at any age. I think plastic surgery is a recognized part of taking care of yourself. It's where hair color was twenty years ago.

I feel that I'm at such a crossroads, being more and more successful. I love to be on television. I love not knowing what I'll be doing from day to day. I'd like to do a Broadway show or summer stock. I know that I'll continue to stay in show business—my possibilities are wide open!

Part III

Your Hair After 40

Chapter 8

Color Counts Most Now

"There's no reason why a woman after forty should not have hair looking better than it's ever looked in her life," says trichologist Philip Kingsley. "By choosing the shade she wants, she can have hair looking better than natural." Now hair coloring can be more of a beauty benefit than ever because it helps restore what nature is removing—your natural color. Through the years the number of pigment producers in the hair follicles, just as in skin, declines, causing hair to fade, turn gray, then eventually white. "Graying usually begins in your forties," states Dr. Earle W. Brauer, vice-president of medical affairs at Revlon. "By age fifty, 50 percent of all people are gray. Graying starts at the temples, then the front of the hair. The speed at which it occurs is genetically determined and varies from person to person. And although certain races gray to a lesser degree than others, no race is spared."

The psychological impact of hair color cannot be denied—it's the first thing someone notices about you! "We are identified by the color of our hair," observes Vern Silverman, director of product performance research at Clairol. "You are the redhead, or the blond, or the one with the white streak. And I think the first thing people look at if they are trying to determine your age is how gray you are." "Gray hair is not really gray—it's a mix of white or colorless hair and the existing natural color. It can be the result of aging, of serious illness, sudden shock, or a lack of any number of minerals and vitamins," explains Leland Hirsch, director of hair color at Nubest & Co. Salon, Manhasset, New York, and special consultant to Clairol, New Product Development. "Hair color is an inherited characteristic, determined by melanin, the main coloring pigment. Beginning as a colorless substance, melanin first turns black through enzyme action, then as pigment granules form into different shapes and sizes, the larger granules become darker hair, while the smaller ones become lighter hair. Graying occurs when there is a lack of activity in the cells preventing the formation of melanin."

Your hair coloring works with your skin coloring—as hair loses pigment and turns gray, skin loses color. Think of it as nature's way of maintaining color balance. You can see the extent of the change if you return to your childhood hair color—it will be too dark for your current skin tone, intensifying your features and actually playing up lines and wrinkles. "Lighter hair color softens the complexion and the features," points out Leland. "And it's important to limit extreme contrasts between hair and skin color now; the face after forty demands a more subtle image."

So whether you decide to cover your gray or flaunt it, there are a multitude of techniques that allow you to do both so naturally that only you—or your hairdresser—will know for sure!

As you age, your hair grows more slowly—this is part of the general, overall, and inevitable growth slowdown—and thins slightly. For most women, though, especially those with colored hair, this does not seem to present a problem, because color helps to thicken hair. Hair volume depends not only on the number of hairs you have but also on the dimension of the hair strand itself. For example, although natural blondes have fine hairs, they have a lot of them—more in fact than anyone else—and about fifty thousand more than redheads. While redheads have fewer hairs, each of their hairs is thicker, so that their head of hair looks just as full, or fuller. Coarse hair is thicker than fine hair, and curly hair is generally thicker than straight hair. "By the time any woman is fifty, though, she'll have finer hair than at twenty," explains Philip Kingsley. "This thinning process is terribly gradual and fractional and started long before she was forty, even though that's the age when, perhaps becoming more critical of herself, she looks in the mirror and thinks—'Oh my God, what's happened to my hair!'"

Now, you want to put back what time may be taking away, but color is only part of the process. The way you wear your hair and the care you give it also helps restore its radiance. "Coloring swells the hair shaft, giving it body but making it more likely to break, so you have to use moisturizers and conditioners to keep it healthy," advises Kingsley. A healthy scalp and head of hair insures that color holds and lasts the way it is supposed to. A great cut and style then maximizes your color impact and complements your total look. More about cut and condition in the chapters that follow.

CHANGING YOUR HAIR COLOR

Each of your hairs is made up of three layers—the cuticle, the cortex, and the medulla. The *cuticle*, or outer layer, consists of keratin—the same fibrous protein that forms skin's outer layer—in overlapping cells, like shingles on a roof. These protect the core of the hair and guard against moisture loss; hair, like skin, needs water to remain elastic and supple. The *cortex*, which lies directly inside the cuticle, contains the pigment granules that determine hair color. The *medulla*, or innermost layer, is a bit of a mystery. Not much is known about its function except that hair can still be healthy even if it's fragmented or missing.

Temporary rinses involve the cuticle alone—they deposit color over it. Semipermanent products do the same; they penetrate the hair strand as well, but certainly not as much as permanent solutions that alter hair's chemical structure, penetrating the cuticle so that the cells lift, then entering the cortex to remove or add color to it.

Because the outer layer is roughened slightly, the hair strand feels thicker and hair looks fuller. The closer the color you choose is to your natural shade, the fewer chemicals you need to achieve it, so the easier the process is on your hair. Also, the more it will work with your skin, eyes, and eyebrow color. "When selecting a hair color, consider not only your natural color, but your complexion, eye color, and the amount of graying or fading that's taken place," advises Leland Hirsch, who offers the following chart as a guide:

HAIR COLOR GOALS FOR THE WOMAN OVER FORTY

Natural Hair Color

Com-plexion Tones	Black–Dk Brown–Med Brown	Lt Brown–Dk Blond–Med Blond	Natural Blond	Natural Red
	All Eye Colors	**All Eye Colors**	**All Eye Colors**	**All Eye Colors**
Olive (green)	FADING: Use the same shade as own natural hair color to brighten drabness.	FADING: Enrich hair color to a slightly deeper tone.	FADING AND GRAYING: Deepen hair with toned-down shades of ash blond.	FADING AND GRAYING: Keep hair in its natural color range, but tone it down slightly.
	GRAYING: Enrich gray with medium ash-brown tones.	GRAYING: Enrich hair color to a slightly deeper tone.		
Sallow (yellow)	FADING: Use warm tones like auburn and dark golden brown *plus* aubergine (wine-plum) tones.	FADING: Brighten with highlights or add lively golden-reddish tones.	FADING: Brighten blond tones with gold and yellow-blond.	FADING: Perk up reds with more intensity.
	GRAYING: Use warm tones like auburn and dark golden browns.	GRAYING: Blend gray with warm tones, maintaining natural color and adding a minimum amount of highlighting.	GRAYING: Lighten dark strands to tones of natural hair color. Deepen gray to natural blond color, keeping overall tone ashy.	GRAYING: Blend gray with subtle red tones.

HAIR COLOR GOALS FOR THE WOMAN OVER FORTY

Natural Hair Color

Com- plexion Tones	Black–Dk Brown– Med Brown All Eye Colors	Lt Brown–Dk Blond–Med Blond All Eye Colors	Natural Blond All Eye Colors	Natural Red All Eye Colors
Ruddy (pink)	FADING: Lighten hair to lighter tones of golden brown and red brown *plus* plum and red tones.	FADING AND GRAYING: Add auburn, red, or gold tones; lighten to brighten gray; highlight to blend natural gray.	FADING: Brighten hair with golden and strawberry blond tones.	FADING: Brighten color with rich red tones.
	GRAYING: Lighten hair to lighter tones of golden brown.		GRAYING: Enrich gray to natural color or to warm golden blond tones.	GRAYING: Blend gray while enriching natural redness.
Neutral (beige)	FADING: Using same shade as own natural color or one shade lighter, lift drabness with just a hint of gold.	FADING AND GRAYING: Frosting, streaking, and highlighting work well—as does any lighter tone.	FADING AND GRAYING: Either lighten hair a full shade or stay in the natural color range, using ash or beige tones.	FADING: Enrich tone back to natural color or intensify it.
	GRAYING: Enrich gray with warm brown tones.			GRAYING: Blend gray to natural red tones and intensify the red.

YOUR HAIR COLOR GLOSSARY

You've probably heard the terms but may not fully understand the differences between them. Basically, all coloring formulas—for both professional and at-home use—fall into two categories: those that wash out and those that don't.

Hair color that washes out

This category includes both temporary and semipermanent color. Neither change the structure of the hair, but by depositing color onto the hair strand, they add body and fullness.

• *Temporary rinses*—provide tone more than actual color; last from shampoo to shampoo.

• *Semipermanent colors*—add highlights and luster but do not lighten dark hair; are really long-lasting rinses that fade gradually after four to eight shampoos. If you apply semipermanent color very often, color builds up to such a degree that it will not wash out.

• *Henna*—this natural plant substance coats the hair strand and gradually fades away. Like semipermanent color, it will become permanent if it's used often enough. Pure henna colors hair red, black henna darkens hair, and neutral henna is believed to add body. Results are unpredictable, though, and a more detailed discussion of henna follows later in this chapter.

Hair color that does not wash out

This category includes tints and double process color, involving bleaching as a first step, that penetrate the cortex of each hair to remove or alter its pigment. These products require premixing of two solutions or a solution and a powder and usually contain ammonia as the active ingredient that causes cuticle cells to rise. Color lasts until it grows out, and new regrowth has to be retouched.

• *Double process color*—this is the procedure that transforms brunettes into pale blondes. Because the color change is so dramatic, you first have to remove the existing color ("bleaching" or "stripping" used to be the terms, but now companies refer to the procedure as "prelightening"), then apply the new color, called the "toner," separately. Since this process removes hair farthest from its natural color, it needs the most maintenance.

• *Single process color*—also called "tinting," this process covers and blends gray, and allows you to go a few shades lighter; the lightening and coloring action are achieved in one step.

• *Highlighting, frosting, streaking*—are the most natural-looking blonding methods because only selected strands of the hair are lightened. Although the terms are often interchanged, *frosting*, explains Leland Hirsch, is when hair is finely woven (selected strands of hair are lifted out with the end of a rattail comb—a procedure referred to as "weaving"), then bleached to a pale blond or white stage. When done correctly, frosting doesn't need to be followed with a toner. *Highlighting* also involves weaving hair finely, but the bleach used is milder and left on hair for a shorter time so that hair is bleached to warmer gold shades. These blend with the natural color to create a more natural look than frosting. You don't need a toner because you're using the natural pigments of the hair to provide the tone. *Streaking* is the process where hair not woven as finely contrasts browns and blonds to create color effects. The degree of bleaching depends on the tones that will blend best with hair's natural color.

If you've already been coloring your hair for years and it no longer looks or feels like hair, before doing anything else, run, don't walk, to the best expert you know for correction of damage. If you don't know who to ask, Clairol has set up a telephone hot line, which is toll-free, to answer questions about hair color and care: 1-800-223-5800. (If you live in New York State, call collect: 1-212-644-2990.)

MAINTAINING GRAY

While gray hair may not be for every woman, it may look marvelous on you. "Women who gray quickly, whose hair becomes close to being very white in just a few years, often keep it that way," says Vern Silverman. So, if you like your gray hair, by all means keep it. "But keep it shiny," advises Leland Hirsch. "Keep it rich—anywhere from white to deep silver, without any yellow or blue or violet. Gray hair can look dull and dry if it's not maintained properly."

Maintenance includes a temporary rinse or semipermanent product to liven the color. Hirsch suggests neutral shades like ash, when you want to keep the same tone, or silver, when you want to deepen the gray. He cautions against platinum hues, which give hair an unnatural bluish cast. If you have a good amount of gray distributed unevenly throughout your hair, frosting in highlights or lighter streaks to blend in with the white hairs can be an alternative. Adds Vern, "Gray in excess of 50 percent can look aging, but frosting in streaks on the very same head tends to change the perception of both the woman who has it done and the person who views it. When the gray is out of a bottle, it becomes an elegant look instead of an aging one."

SHOULD YOU OR SHOULDN'T YOU COLOR YOUR HAIR YOURSELF?

"There are women who like to do their own color, just as there are those who don't feel they can—they don't want to take the responsibility," states Vern Silverman. "They like going to a salon for the entire treatment, not only the coloring. They want someone to wash their hair, cut it, groom it, and maintain it. Yet I've seen beautiful work done at home. A lot of women get good results when they do their color with a friend."

Basically, whether or not you should color your hair yourself depends upon your budget, schedule, and hair needs: the simpler the coloring procedure, the simpler and less expensive it is to do yourself. Adds Vern, "You can go into the bathroom and put on your coloring—twenty-five minutes later, it's finished and you are free for the next month."

Some women view professional coloring as an indulgence, others, a necessity, but if you have the means, the time, or the need for it, the effects can be quite astonishing. Said one woman about her colorist, "I think it's important to keep a list of experts in every field—makeup, fashion, hair, fitness, even plastic surgery—people whose advice I can trust to guide me. But these have to be the best, because I believe I should always try to give myself the best!"

If trips to the beauty salon do not fit into your schedule or budget, yet you want your hair to have every advantage, consider a coloring technique that requires little salon maintenance, like highlighting, or invest in a consultation and initial coloring session with an expert to work out a program that you can continue at home; most colorists are very happy to oblige.

HOW TO FIND A GOOD COLORIST

While you might be able to find the right hair stylist by asking a woman whose cut you admire who does her hair, the same is not true for color. Color that's obvious is *not* what you want, so go ahead and ask the color-

ist's name, but only so you can avoid him or her.

Word of mouth is one of the best ways of finding a competent colorist, asking friends and acquaintances if they can recommend someone, then going into the salon for a consultation to see what can be done for your hair and to view his or her work in progress. You're seeking a trained expert—someone with a wonderful color sense as well as technical skill. You can also look through the pages of the fashion and beauty magazines at the credits or write to the beauty editors or reader service departments for a list of experts in your area.

HAIR COLOR A COLORIST WOULD DO

What would a leading professional actually do to your hair right now? Leland Hirsch talks about the ways that he would use color to offset graying and fading and to restore hair's richness and luster, and offers pointers that you can discuss with your colorist or perhaps try at home yourself.

Leland likes to stay within the natural color range of the hair, using tones that lighten and brighten what is already there. After forty, he says, when you have a high percentage of gray, darker colors are not only unflattering but are impractical, too, since they make roots all the more apparent—hair grows in every three to four weeks. Semipermanent hair color is his way of dealing with a small percentage of gray; it enriches the natural color and adds depth and tone without lightening.

When using tints or semipermanent color on salt-and-pepper hair, the best, most natural effect is blending—lightening the darker hairs and darkening the lighter ones so that the two never meet, but approach each other. He strives for variation rather than coverage, which looks unnatural. Blending does not require much touching up, and hair grows in without a marked line. But this particular process is an art and really has to be performed by a professional: it involves a mix of two or three shades, precisely applied.

When hair is naturally dark brown or black, he moves to the deep aubergine and wine colors. When it's naturally red, beginning to gray or lose pigment so that it gets deeper or lighter, he moves toward the reddish-gold tones, as less intense reds make new gray growth appear as soft highlights. When naturally blond hair tends to grow either darker or lighter through the years, he livens the color. With graying blondes he likes semipermanent color in golden tones; with darkening blondes he'll use a tint to lighten.

Another solution for correcting darkening or lightening hair that's medium-to-very-light blond is lightening with foil. Hair that's subtly highlighted can be worn in any style, but when highlights are more apparent, hair should not be cut close and layered, because it will look choppy.

If you are considering henna, Leland advises against it, for several reasons. "I just don't find it healthy for hair. It's a natural ingredient, imported to this country, and tends to collect bacteria." Another negative—unpredictability: Red henna turns gray hair orange, while dark and neutral henna can turn gray and light hair green. "I also have found that instead of adding body—a plus many attribute to henna—it dries hair out and weighs it down."

HAIR COLORING YOU CAN DO

Naturally, the least complicated coloring process is the easiest to do yourself: the least time-consuming, the least expensive. And if you stay within your natural color range—as our expert suggests—you'll have little problem with regrowth, saving your hair wear and tear. One of the great advantages of graying is that you can keep your hair color lighter with little effort since it's naturally lighter to begin with.

For all but the most temporary colors, though, the experts recommend a patch test for allergies and a preview test to see how the color "takes" on your hair. Even when the process is not permanent, you want to avoid unsightly mistakes, and since the color shown on the box is often the way it would look on pure white hair, you won't know how it will look on your hair until you try it. Give yourself these tests at the same time, about twenty-four hours before you've scheduled your coloring session.

• *The patch test*—allergies can develop suddenly; you can be irritated this week by an ingredient that did not bother you last week, so a patch test before every coloring session is a good idea. Prepare about a tablespoonful of your test mixture. Wash an area about the size of a quarter on the inside of your elbow with a mild soap and water; pat dry. Apply a few drops of the product to this area

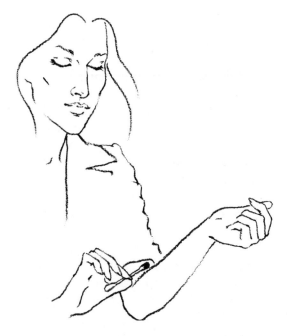

with a cotton swab. Leave the area uncovered for twenty-four hours. Any reddening, burning, itching, or irritation in or around the test area indicates an allergic reaction. If there is no reaction, you are not allergic to the mixture and can proceed.

• *The preview test*—the interaction between your natural color and the color you see on the box will determine the color you get. Test this color by snipping a swatch of hair, about a quarter-inch wide and the entire length of the hair strands (if you are concerned about how your gray areas will look, snip a swatch that includes both gray and your natural color), then taping this swatch together at the roots. Dip it into the remaining test mixture, making sure that it is saturated, and wait about twenty to twenty-five minutes for the color to take, then wipe the swatch clean with a damp towel. Check the color. If it's not the shade you want, return the swatch to the mixture (provided its coloring action does not shut off automatically after a certain time) until it is the right shade. If it's still wrong, try a different color. As soon as you arrive at the color or intensity you like, and when your patch test proves negative, go ahead with your coloring. You may find the following tips helpful as well, when you're doing your color yourself or with a friend:

• Set up your mirrors so that you have a clear view of the back and the sides of your hair. You don't want to apply color blindly.

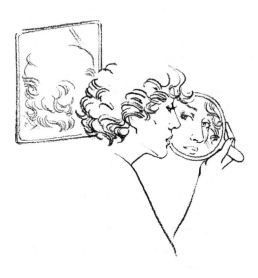

• Check product directions beforehand to learn what tools you'll need—a bowl, cotton, timer, and so on. Assemble everything so there won't be any last-minute interference.

• Protect the skin around your hairline with a film of petroleum jelly.

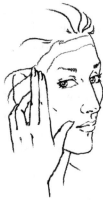

• Don't use coloring directly after a permanent; it's best to wait a few weeks.

• Treat your hair and scalp gently. Don't comb or brush excessively; avoid irritation that would contribute to scalp sensitivity.

• Follow all instructions—including timing—to the letter.

• With permanent colors, prepare the mixture immediately before use and keep at room temperature. Never keep any leftover mixture, because the container can burst.

• Use a plastic rather than metal comb.

• Apply color at the crown, working toward the nape. Do the front last. It will look more natural this way; plus, chemicals—which can be damaging when left on too long—stay on the shortest amount of time.

• Wear plastic gloves to protect your skin when applying color.

Now you are ready for the effects you can create and the ways to go about them. Although the exact directions differ from product to product, the following information can give you a fast idea of the amount of work that goes into each coloring technique:

• *For temporary highlights, or to try on a tone*—a temporary rinse will intensify your natural color and mask yellow in gray hair. Color washes out in your next shampoo. First shampoo hair, then towel it dry; apply rinse to still-damp hair. Leave in for about one-half hour, then rinse with warm water.

• *For richness and sheen, to blend gray or enhance or lift your natural color*—a semipermanent formulation will give you richer highlights than a temporary rinse, yet provide color that you don't have to live with very long—it will eventually wash out. Since results are always a bit darker than the package indicates, select a shade lighter than your hair. You have a choice between foam or lotion. To apply either one, you first section your dry hair, then apply color a

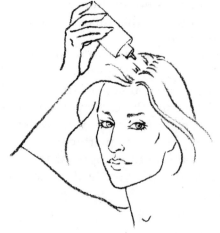

little at a time. After you've distributed the entire contents throughout your hair, work it into a lather, covering all hair without rubbing the formulation into your

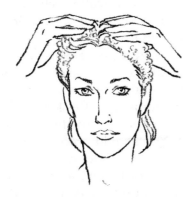

scalp. Put a plastic cap over your saturated hair and leave color on

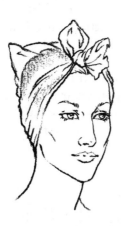

from 20 to 45 minutes. Gray hair tends to be more color resistant; you'll be able to get a better idea about timing from your preview test. Then remove the pastic, add warm water to hair, and work up a rich lather. Rinse. Remember, if you use a semipermanent product very often, the color will build up over the hair strand. Because you want to keep the ends lighter for the most natural re-

sults, after a while apply color to hair roots and regrowth only.

• *For red highlights*—some colorists say they get very pretty results from pure henna on hair that's hardly gray. Henna, though, is a very messy procedure—it's almost like applying a mud pack. If you want to take the chance—and results are unstable—you have to mix the henna powder with hot water and brush it onto clean dry hair that's divided into sections. When you have covered your entire head, comb through the hair with a wide-tooth comb to distribute the henna evenly. Wrap your head in aluminum foil, with a coil of cotton around your hairline to absorb any dripping, and sit under a hairdryer for about

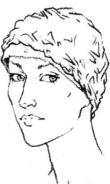

an hour. Rinse henna out with warm water, shampoo hair and scalp thoroughly, and condition the hair. Henna should never be used on previously colored hair or on freshly permed hair; it does not combine well with other processes.

• *For lightening hair several shades and covering gray*—if you have a lot of gray, you'll find that a semipermanent product will not give you enough coverage, so you may need a tint. These are available in shampoo-in formulations as well as lotions, which are first mixed, then applied like a semipermanent product. If you are under 50 percent gray, use your natural color as your color base and select a shade slightly lighter; if you are over 50 percent gray, use gray as your color base, choosing a shade that matches or is lighter. If you go darker, you'll find the final effect too heavy and your regrowth too obvious. However, it can work if hair is left lighter around your face. When retouching, apply color to roots only to avoid an unnatural color buildup on hair ends.

• *For complete color change to produce the palest shades of blond and certain reds when your hair is darker*—you have to bleach hair to remove the existing color and lighten it uniformly, then apply the color you want separately. Double process coloring demands constant upkeep—and caution. If it's done too often, it can damage your hair. Since the color you get will probably be out of the range of your natural color, the results may be less believable than other methods. A more natural, easier-to-maintain way to look blond is through highlighting, the lightening technique favored by the leading hair colorists.

• *For paler streaks and highlights, and an overall blond, gold, even red, richness*—the answer is highlighting. The secret behind the best-looking highlighting is avoiding great contrasts of color and scattering a variety of tones thinly and at random over the head. There are kits that allow you to frost, tip, streak, even finger-paint, your hair yourself, but results will be better if you have a friend help. Even so, it's difficult to achieve the fabulous results of a top-notch professional.

Frosting involves precise timing and cautious experimentation. Streaks should be very slim, in varying intensities: the longer you leave on the bleach, the lighter they will get. You should proceed slowly; you can always add more streaks where you need them. Although the cap in a frosting kit is designed to minimize mistakes, you can't really see which strands of hair you are lightening, so you might want to try the foil method, used by professional colorists. Start by cutting the foil into oblong pieces about four by six inches. Comb your dry hair into the style you wear it, and beginning at the front of your hair, pick up a thin row of hair with the end of a

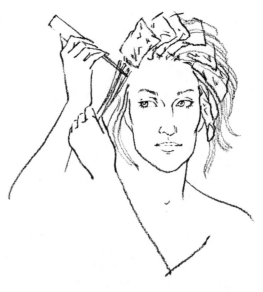

rattail comb, holding the foil underneath it. Brush on bleach, then seal the foil by folding it over. Avoiding

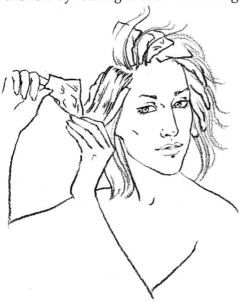

your hairline and part, space rows about a half inch apart. Clip hair that's not being streaked to the foil above it. When you've finished, remove the foil on your first hair strand and scrape off the bleach. You want your hair to look pale and golden. If it's orange, apply more bleach, fold the foil, and check five minutes later. When strands are pale, remove bleach from each strand with warm water, then shampoo your hair and condition it. Frosting needs infrequent retouching—once every three to five months, depending upon your natural color—and looks best on hair that's no darker than medium brown.

Chapter 9

Ageless Hairstyling

"It's a big mistake for a woman to think that because she's getting older, her hair has to be short. It can be any length," states stylist Stephen Jacobs, with New York City's Pierre Michel salon. "It's the line of the hair that is important—the most flattering will be one that 'lifts' her features." Adds free-lance stylist Hugh Harrison, "Hairdos that turn softly back off the face can achieve the effect of a face lift—visually pulling the eye area."

"I've noticed with my clients that by the time a woman has reached forty, she's arrived at a length and a style that becomes her look, and then we simply do extensions on that look," says Stephen Jacobs. "I think every fall a woman should strive for a slight new feeling in her hair, a subtle change that works with the current fashions. It gives a new outlook, makes her feel younger and fresher. People around her notice and are stimulated by it so that they see her in a different way." It's essential to keep your style up to date, advises this expert, but not avant-garde. "The look of the moment should be softened a little," he continues. "Hair, makeup, and fashion move together. The woman with ageless great looks incorporates what's new in her appearance, but adapts it so that it works uniquely for her."

"Two telltale signs you want to avoid are unnatural color and too stiff a hairstyle—one with every hair rigidly in place, then sprayed to stay there. It no longer looks natural or young. Even when hair is coiffed, the effect should be freer, hair should seem touchable," he says. "And good color with no style is worthless. Hair is the first thing you can do something about. Improve its color, its cut, its quality, and you'll feel better about yourself; it's immediate gratification!"

So, your hairdresser may be just as important for your head as a psychiatrist. For while you can color, condition, and maintain your hair yourself, you should definitely put yourself in expert hands for your cut, because everything else you do is dependent upon it.

DETERMINING YOUR BEST LOOK

The shape of your hair begins with the cut you get. Your stylist can actually cut in more curl—important if your hair is thinning, so it will look thicker—or even cut some out, when graying causes your hair to become unruly or less pliable. And while it depends on what your hair can and cannot do, its thickness and texture and its degree of curl, there's more that goes into your best look:

• *Balance for the face*—"We look at face shape in relation to hairstyle differently now," explains Stephen. "We used to try to make everything into a perfect oval, but now we try to create a focal point by emphasizing the best facial qualities." He advises taking your major clue from your eyes—looking to see if they need opening or closing, pulling up or down and then examining your bone structure, and what you want to correct. For example, a round face needs straighter lines to extend the face up and out, not curls that will make it look rounder, while an angular face can carry a curlier, wavier style. "A young girl with prominent bones can look sensational with her straight and angled hair, but the forty-year-old with great bones tends to look hard and harsh with the same hairstyle," he adds.

• *The overall effect*—the length and width of your hair has to balance your height and body type. A close-cropped head is not harmonious with a tall, fleshy frame, while long, voluminous tresses can be overwhelming on a tiny body.

• *Your hair needs*—do you have the kind of hair that goes from wet to dry without a roller? Can you handle your hair yourself? Do you have lots of time to fuss with your look?

• *Your life-style*—is there a certain way you have to look for your job or personal life? The way you live your life can put restrictions on the kind of hairstyle you'll want.

"Hairstyles can be a little more inventive now than they were in the past," explains Stephen Jacobs. "We want to create an effect instead of simply a balanced look—that can be boring. This effect should never be freakish or bizarre. It should just make hair look special. A woman does not want to stand out that much, but she does want to look great."

Of course, there is no one style best for a particular face. You can wear anything, as long as it looks good! However, the complexion and facial changes that influenced your choice of hair color influence your hairstyle too. And this is most important if you have gray hair. Unless it's fashionable, it can look aging and matronly. "Any style that is too structured, too hard on the features, is not complimentary at this point of life; strong lines are not flattering," states Michael Mazzei, owner of Nubest & Co. salon. "If you don't have a wave in your hair, you should consider it. It not only makes hair soft and stylish—the way it should be after forty—it makes it versatile, too. Waves never look the same two days in a row."

HAIR SHAPES THAT "CORRECT" FACIAL CHANGES

Just as you can use your hairstyle to

emphasize your good features, it likewise serves to downplay your bad ones, the changes in your face that often accompany maturity. "You should be interested in creating a feeling with your hairstyle, an illusion," explains Stephen Jacobs, who devised the following looks to show you some of the ways the lines, the shape of your hair, can offset change. "People don't really see all the faults someone has, they get an overall effect, and that's what we want to accomplish with your hairstyle."

These shapes, however, are just suggestions and should not be duplicated line for line. The look you arrive at, after discussion with your stylist, depends on your hair—what it will and will not do—as well as on everything else discussed earlier.

• If you have a lined or furrowed forehead, a feathered bang or a tousled front will hide it. Of course, so will a full bang, but it can be too heavy and overwhelming for the forty-plus face; a soft, wispy fringe is newer, lighter.

• If you have crow's-feet, a shorter, curly look tends to detract from lines around the eyes by providing movement. A hairdo that's straight only extends facial lines.

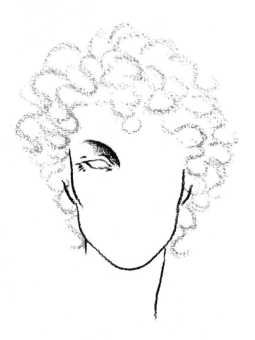

• If you have a sagging jawline, short hair with a longer neckline draws attention away from your jaw. Style hair back at the sides and brush it onto the neck to fill in this area and make it look longer and more tapered.

• If your chin is beginning to recede a bit, balance it with volume and fullness in the front of your hair. This shape draws everything up and away from the chin.

• If your nose is becoming more prominent, or drooping, balance this with height and soft waves. You want to provide a wavy, non-symmetrical frame around the face so that the nose seems absorbed into it.

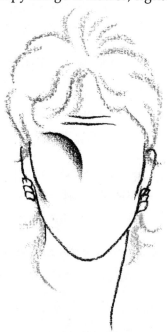

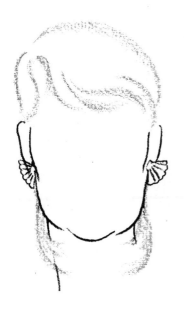

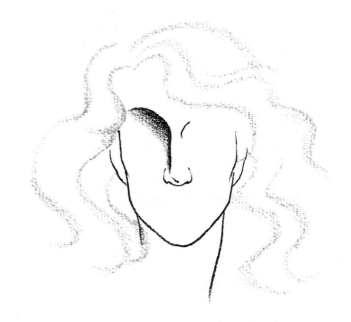

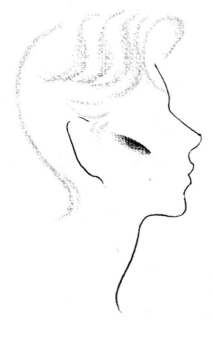

• If your ears seem bigger (wrinkled skin, lengthened earlobes) or if you want to hide any scars from a face lift, try a pageboy with a slightly broken or lifted wave at each ear, so the line of the hair doesn't drag features down and ears are veiled but not hidden.

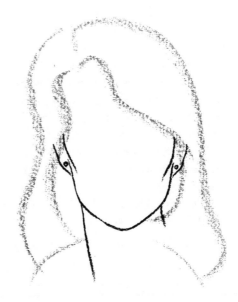

• If your face is thin or thinning, a cut that's layered all over the head, then styled with fullness, will balance a thin or gaunt face.

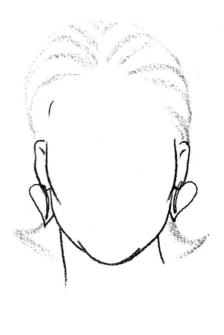

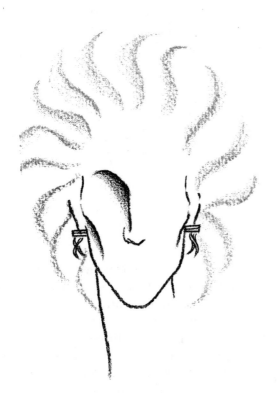

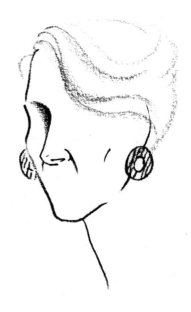

• If your face looks fuller, fleshier, or droopier, keep sides tight and top full and soft to pick facial lines up without adding width.
• If you have prominent folds from nose to mouth, open up your face with a higher, waved front and crown and draw sides back into a soft French twist.

• If your face is angular and becoming more so, a wispy, slightly layered look, where sides are feathered so they break onto the face, will soften your bone structure.

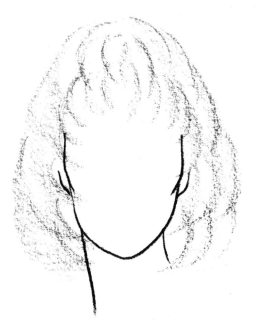

QUICK-CHANGING YOUR LOOK

What can you do when you have a look that basically becomes you, but you want variations on the theme? Here are a few ideas to consider that can add new interest to hair at any length. Remember, though, any change in your hair should be accompanied by one in both makeup and jewelry—your earrings alone can add further appeal to a hairstyle. When your hair is swept away from your face, your makeup will need a revamping—heightened color, perhaps, with more definition around the eyes.

By changing a part, or putting one where you had none, you can look quite different, no matter what your hair length. If your tresses are layered, short, and curly, try for a smoother shape. If they are straighter, add curl via electric rollers or a permanent. Straight hair that's cut one length can gain variety with a body perm for volume, or a partial perm, at the ends, for wave. Wispy bangs pulled onto the forehead are an alternative to hair that's always been pushed back off the brow—they also draw attention to the eyes. If you've been wearing bangs for a while, brush them off your face and see how that looks.

With longer hair you have even more styling options, because aside from the obvious ones—a body wave for straighter hair, with sides angled for softness or caught back with a comb; brushing and blow-drying wavier hair smooth but leaving curve at the sides—you can put hair up in a soft knot, roll, twist, even braid. You don't want to pull your hair severely back, though, unless your face is extraordinary, reminds Stephen Jacobs, as most faces after forty need a soft frame. You can also enhance your hair with hairpieces—as an ornament, a braid perhaps to wrap around a chignon or a filler; a switch of hair to fill a French twist or a roll—but stay away from obvious wigs or falls. Speak to your hairdresser about the add-ons that will work for you, and let him or her show you how to use them.

FINDING A HAIR STYLIST

Asking a woman with hair similar to yours, in a style you like, who cuts her hair is certainly a valid way to find a competent hair stylist, as long as you don't assume that you can have exactly the same look. There are a multitude of factors involved in creating a hairdo—and hair type is only one of them. You can also ask friends and acquaintances to recommend a stylist, then schedule a consultation or, better, a styling session, so you can see how your hair is handled, and the stylist can see how your hair moves and reacts. Make an appointment for a cut when you are satisfied that the stylist understands your hair and your needs. Additional ways are querying the woman's editor of your local newspaper, who probably is familiar with experts in your area, and writing to the beauty editor of your favorite magazine for names. If you know about someone wonderful in another city, maybe it's time for a vacation—to see the sights and schedule a haircut. When you return home, your local stylist can follow the lines of the new cut.

TALKING TO YOUR HAIR STYLIST

You can't get what you want if you don't tell your stylist what that is—creating a great look is a joint venture. Stephen Jacobs says that honesty is essential. Be truthful about what you want your hairstyle to do. A lot of experts find it's easier to understand what a client means if she has pictures. So clip the looks you like when you see them in magazines, but realize that many can't be duplicated. Some styles are created only for the photograph and are not practical for real life. Also, allow yourself to be interviewed. Discuss the fashions you like to wear, the time you have for your hair, the places you go, the amount of effort you're willing to put into your look. Then stand up; your stylist will most likely ask you to—to check your height and body type. As you know, they both figure into your final hairstyle.

The real test of a good cut, however, is when you get home, after the first shampoo you give yourself—the moment when you have to re-create the look.

SALON TECHNIQUES YOU CAN DO—SETTING

There are certain salon methods that you can easily do at home, like setting with a brush and blow-dryer, with rollers, pin curls, or a curling iron, not to mention permanent waving. And even if you are one of the lucky ones who can go from wet to dry without a comb, there still may be moments when you want a little more curve or curl or finish to your hairdo, and that's when setting can help.

Setting with a brush and blow-dryer

You'll learn the best way to blow-dry for fullness in the next chapter. Here's how to "set" and style your hair with a round bristle brush—the thinner the brush, the tighter the curl. A thicker brush is good for waves and overall fullness. When your hair is dried to damp, roll small, neat sections of it around the brush in the direction you want your curl or wave to go. Then hold the dryer over each section for a few seconds, letting hair cool in the brush before unwinding. Never focus the dryer's direct heat on one spot for too long. Work up the back of the head to the crown, then the crown from back to front. If your hair is very short, or if you don't want curl, catch a section of it at a time in a plastic wide-bristle brush and pull gently in the opposite direction hair is to fall; dry; then realign hair in the direction it's supposed to go. When finished, ruffle

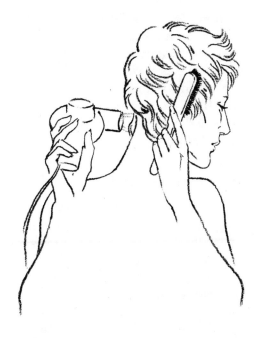

your hair with your fingers and smooth ends with a comb. For added shape, flick ends up or under with a curling iron or electric rollers.

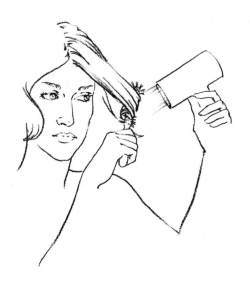

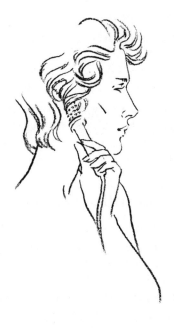

No matter what your hair length or style, you should never overdry it. To avoid damage and breakage, many experts recommend that you stop drying your hair while it still has a little moisture left in it, allowing it to dry on its own for the next few minutes.

Setting with rollers

Hairstyles that need lift and body can get both with a roller setting. It's especially advisable on frizzy, bleached hair because blow-drying can turn it to straw, but roller setting can smooth it. The larger the roller used, the larger the wave or curl; the smaller the roller, the tighter the curl. The disadvantage in roller setting lies in the time it takes to roll your hair and then to dry it.

You can roll your hair when it's very wet, or save time by letting it dry naturally, then rewetting hair about half an inch from the roots before rolling it. To avoid crimped or frazzled ends, use setting papers, then wind hair smoothly in mesh, plastic, or sponge rollers, and dry hair. The set will look more natural if you blow-dry hair roots after you remove the rollers, then brush hair thoroughly so hair loses any stiffness.

Setting with heated rollers

A heated-roller set is a time-saver—it provides instant wave and curl and can also smooth and tame frizzy or bushy hair, but the set does not last as long as one with regular rollers or pin curls. When you're shopping for heated rollers, select a set

with a variety of roller sizes to meet all of your setting needs, and spikes that are not sharp. If you travel, a dual-voltage set makes sense.

When you're rolling your hair, remember that the curl takes best on hair that's freshly shampooed and almost dry. You should try a test curl to time your set and see just how much curl you get: the amount depends on the size of the roller and the length of time you leave it in—a larger roller left in hair a shorter time will give the loosest, easiest wave. For maximum volume, leave rollers in hair until they have cooled completely. When winding your hair around the roller, use setting paper. It keeps ends smooth and protects them from too much heat. Use a small amount of hair on each roller and wind in the direction you want the curl or wave to go. Wind the

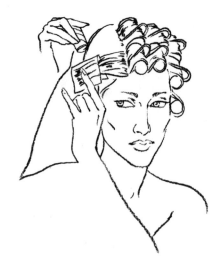

roller snugly but without pulling your hair. Unwind the rollers carefully—especially now, when every hair counts—working from the bottom of the head to the crown. As you unwind, pin each curl into place. When the entire head is cool, comb or brush hair into the style you want. But you don't always have to set your entire head; you can just wind a few rollers in the spots you need them. Try not to overuse heated rollers, because they can ultimately dry hair out. If you find that happening, consider a permanent or a new hairstyle that needs less maintenance to look good.

Setting with pin curls

You can pin-curl your whole head for a very curly do, or pin-curl in places to keep the line of a style. In fact, you'll often see the latter done

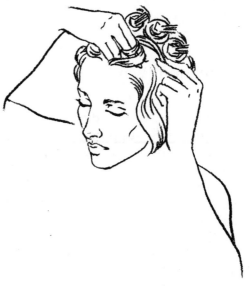

in the beauty salon—after hair is styled with a brush and blow-dryer. Wind a pin curl by wrapping a thin section of hair around one, two, or

three fingers in the direction you want the curl to go. Then catch it into a flat curl and anchor it with a bobby pin or clip in the inside only. The more fingers you wind your hair around, the larger the pin curl. A pin curl gives a tighter, closer-to-the-roots curl than one set with a roller.

Setting with a curling iron

These magic wands are wonderful for adding fullness and form exactly where you want it—around the face or on hair ends. Do not use them on fragile and damaged hair, because the concentrated heat they provide is too strong. Look for a lightweight iron coated with Teflon or plastic and temperature controlled by a built-in thermostat. It's best to leave the professional-type curling iron to the professional, since it gets very hot and needs expert handling.

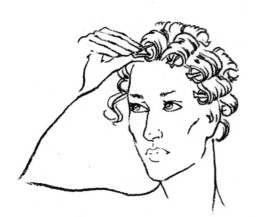

Use a curling iron on dry hair only, winding small sections of hair at a time and testing your hair after several seconds to see how quickly it curls. After you unwind the curl, pin it in place and let it cool completely before you comb your hair.

Permanent wave setting

"Weak-looking hair is aging," says Stephen Jacobs. "Body waves are soft and give support to the hair, creating a stronger, fuller look. They are good for all hair except the thinnest, most fragile." Think of a body wave as a permanent way to set your hair. It alters the structure of the hair so that a new shape is locked in. You can wear hair dried naturally for day and blow-dried and set for a more structured evening look.

Body waves last for several months, depending upon hair growth and the strength of the solution. A straightener operates on the same principle, but instead of adding curl, it takes it away. Unlike the permanents of yore that resulted in a mass of frizz, today's perms, body waves in particular, are buffered with conditioners so that damage is kept to a minimum—even tinted hair can be permed.

As with coloring, perms can be done at home or in a salon. But if you can have a professional give you yours, you should. "An at-home permanent that's too weak is probably worse for your hair than one that's too strong," says Michael Mazzei. "The damage is done even if the results are not what you want. You only compound the problem by redoing the process." The amount of hair rolled on each roll, the tension, the timing, hair sectioning and the manner in which rods are clipped has to be just so. After your permanent, wait at least two days to wash your hair, because the active ingredients in shampoo can loosen the set. Wait at least two weeks after coloring your hair before you perm it, conditioning it frequently; then wait at least one week after your perm to recolor your hair. Don't be surprised if your hair is a shade lighter after a permanent, and remember that permed hair, like colored hair, has to be protected from the sun.

SALON TECHNIQUES YOU CAN DO—STYLING

Backcombing

A light backcombing—where hair is combed in the direction opposite to the one it should go so that it's fluffed up from underneath—can add fullness to any hair look, any length. The secret is to backcomb gently, in small sections, using a fine-tooth rattail comb on hair that's not fragile or in bad condition.

The technique: Beginning at the front of your head, comb a one- to two-inch section of hair straight out from your head. Then, holding the ends in one hand, slide the comb down the hair toward the scalp, using slow, even strokes, so that the section stands out from your head.

If it falls, take a larger section and repeat your actions a little more firmly. When you've backcombed your entire head or the areas of your hair where you want height or

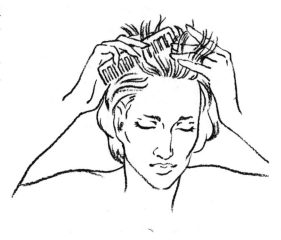

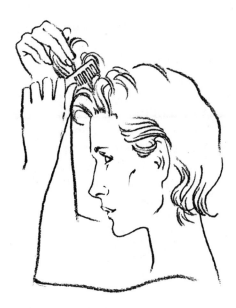

width, smooth a layer of hair over the backcombing to conceal it, with a brush or a comb. Backcombing is most effective if you first shampoo then blow-dry your hair with your head lowered, setting it with electric rollers if it needs more wave.

Removing backcombing: Using a wide-tooth comb, remove backcombing gently, starting at the ends of the hair and working toward the scalp. Never pull your hair, and if there are hard-to-remove tangles, try to separate them with your fingers first or the tail of your fine-tooth

comb. Always take out backcombing before sleeping, because it can cause hair to break.

Twisting

A classic French twist is a wonderfully elegant and feminine look and a perennial favorite. Although it's a bit tricky to do yourself, these hints should make it easier.

Brush all hair to one side of your head and anchor it firmly with a row of bobby pins from your nape to

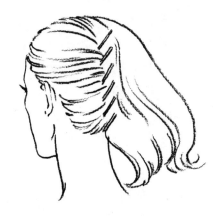

crown. Now brush all hair smooth and twist it over the bobby pins in an upward direction, anchoring it at

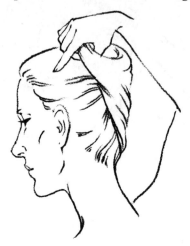

the crown with a hairpin. Then use hairpins or bobby pins to hold the seam of the twist against your head.

You can fashion a full twist or partial ones to keep your hair softly off the sides of your face. Partial twists are easiest if you first dampen the side of your hair from the temple to the ear, hold it taut, and twist it back, anchoring it behind the ear

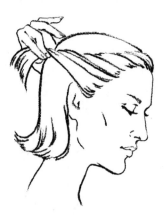

with a bobby pin. Leave the other side loose or twist it, too, then twist the bottom hair into a knot at the nape.

Knotting

A chignon is a chic way to catch all hair back—you can wear one at the nape of your neck, or the crown, and in matter of seconds. Brush all of your hair into a ponytail at the top of your head and fasten it with a coated elastic band. Make sure that your hair is not pulled too tightly; it should be rather loose and full, you can even pull out a few wisps. Comb through the ponytail, then dampen it slightly and twist it tightly, pushing the end into the center of the area held by the elastic band to create a knot. Twist hair ends around and under and anchor with bobby pins or hairpins.

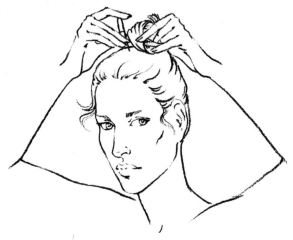

Rolling

Rolling is another longer hair option that lifts the features and nicely frames the face. Begin by combing all hair smooth. If the front of your hair is shorter, leave it loose and tousled; if it's long, try rolling it as well. You should roll your hair in segments from front to back in whatever thickness becomes you. If you want fullness, you probably have to backcomb hair lightly, combing hair over the backcombing so that it is smooth, and then roll it. Now starting at the forehead or in front of the ear, roll your hair in a thick section as pictured and pin the roll in place gently, leaving the ends loose. Take the next section of hair, including the ends, and roll. Pin as you did the previous one. Continue rolling section by section until you reach the nape, leaving ends loose. Roll the other side of your hair beginning at the forehead or behind the ear, in the same way. When you reach the nape, roll the two sets of ends up over your fingers like a fat

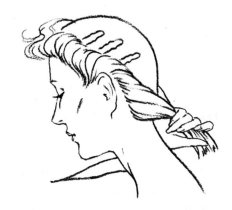

pin curl and pin through the roll to hide it. Anchor the entire roll firmly to the scalp with pins, and pull out wisps if the roll looks too severe.

Chapter 10

Hair Care for Optimum Body

"Don't be worried if your hair is a little drier now; dry hair has more body," explains expert Michael Mazzei. This dryness, the result of a combination of causes including a natural slowdown in oil gland activity, chemical processing, and/or heated appliances, can actually be used to great advantage. Hair can look lusher, thicker, even if it is not, and that's good news.

As Michael points out, "To get more and more body, do less—just keep hair clean, and if it's not manageable, finish with a lightweight conditioner on hair ends only. Deep conditioning, hot oil, for example, will only soften hair and weigh it down, and that's what you don't want." Happily, as you grow older, instead of getting more complicated, hair care becomes even easier. "Gray hair does not have to be treated any differently, unless you're treating a cosmetic deficit," adds Dr. Earle Brauer. "If your hair becomes more difficult to manage because gray hair tends to get wiry, simply condition more frequently." Hair after forty, he continues, is easier to pull out so it has to be treated gently and manipulated as little as possible.

"When talking about hair care, you can't underestimate the importance of your psychological and physical health," stresses Michael. "And exercise is essential to both. It stimulates the blood flow to the scalp, providing nourishment to the hair follicles, and it makes you feel better about yourself. When you feel good, every part of you looks good. In fact, we believe so strongly in the beneficial effects of exercise on hair, that we're including exercise facilities in the salon." True, your hair, like your skin, mirrors your moods and ever-changing body chemistry. "The real secret to corrective and preventive hair care is adjusting your program, your products, to these changes," he continues. "Don't use the same shampoo, the same conditioner consistently. Your hair goes through cycles and has different needs at different times. That's also why your hair-coloring formulation should be frequently adjusted. And when you're in a slump or feel out of sorts or it's that time of the month, your hair shows it, so stay away from chemical processes—coloring, perming—at those times and have your hair shampooed and styled, or get a facial instead."

HAIR-CARE BASICS

Like every other part of you—your attitude, your skin, your shape—

your hair is going through changes. It becomes drier. For some women it seems thinner or finer. Or feels coarser with graying—white hairs are less uniform and regular than those of your natural color, so they don't feel as smooth. "Not only does hair begin to change with hormonal shifts, so that its rate of growth, fall-out, replacement, and diameter are affected, but you're probably also starting to do all the things that are physically traumatic to it," observes Philip Kingsley. Because putting back what nature is taking away involves processes that are very hard on hair, proper care is now more important than ever. It begins with the right kind of combing and brushing, shampooing and conditioning, then proceeds to blow-drying and finally to the best ways of treating hair problems.

COMBING AND BRUSHING

"The concept of brushing for softness and shine is outdated and counterproductive today," says Dr. Earle Brauer, "because friction damages the hair shaft. And it can be catastrophic to hair that's in an already weakened state. You have to reduce the vigor of your handling, not increase it. Think of combing and brushing as grooming techniques—to replace, style, and smooth the hair."

When combing: Detangle your hair—especially before and after shampooing—with a wide-tooth comb. Make sure the teeth are rounded at the tips so they won't

scratch or injure your hair and scalp. Always comb your hair from the

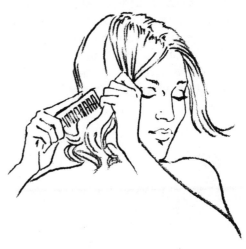

ends up to avoid pulling it. Begin several inches from hair ends and gently run the comb through, working your way gradually toward the crown, combing hair a few inches at a time. If your hair is long or badly snarled, hold ends in one hand while you work with the other through the portion of the hair closest to the roots.

Arrange your hair with an all-purpose comb—one that is divided into a wide- and a narrow-tooth section. Backcomb with a rattail comb—it is also useful when winding rollers.

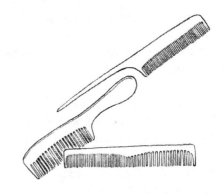

When brushing: Detangle and smooth hair using a flat brush with either wide-tooth plastic bristles, natural bristles if your hair is fine or medium, or a mixture of natural and plastic bristles if your hair is coarser. The brush with wide teeth is also helpful in shaping hair while you blow it dry.

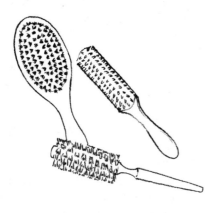

Style your hair when drying it with a round brush. The bristles can be natural or a mixture as long as they are smooth and tapered at the ends, not sharp. The diameter of the brush depends upon your hairstyle—a thinner brush will give a tighter curl.

Cleaning your comb and brush: You should clean your hair tools as often as possible—at least once a week. Soak them for a maximum of ten minutes in a basin of warm water with shampoo or dishwashing liquid, then shake them gently and blot with a towel. Let them dry naturally. If brush bristles are natural, make sure you do not soak them for too long or the bristles can loosen and fall out. Dry the brush away from a direct source of heat.

MASSAGE

Scalp massage can have very soothing effects. Massage relaxes a scalp tightened by tension and stress, and it revs up the blood flow to the scalp, which also tends to slow down through the years. It can likewise stimulate the oil glands to produce more oil, a boon to dry scalps but certainly not to oily ones. You do, however, have to keep your motions gentle and smooth—massaging as if you were shampooing can rub hairs against each other, causing damage to the cuticle layer.

Massage your scalp with the balls of your fingers. Grasp your scalp with your fingers—working from the front to the back of the head—your wrists are arched and fingers remain in one place at a time; work one area completely before moving on to the next, moving or raising them from the scalp, as if you were kneading dough.

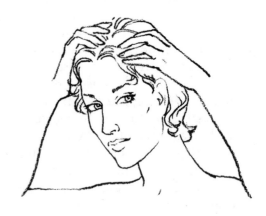

SHAMPOOING

Your hair and scalp should be washed as often as necessary to stay clean and healthy. For many experts, this means daily. "You can wash your hair every day just like your skin," says Dr. Norman Orentreich. "Skin was designed as protection for the body, and hair as protection for the skin. Both require and do better with active cleansing." Adds Philip Kingsley, "Hair always looks best when it's freshly washed, and as a woman grows older she knows this; she knows that glossy hair makes her look better."

With shampooing, as with every other beauty technique, the manner in which it's performed is very important, more so at this time when overmanipulating can add insult to injury. Rinsing is also crucial. Shampoo that's left in your hair can dry and dull it, and irritate your scalp, too. "You can rinse your hair more effectively if you shampoo in the shower," says Michael Mazzei. "Shampoo, rinse, then apply your conditioner and let it work while you soap your body. Finally, rinse everything off at once."

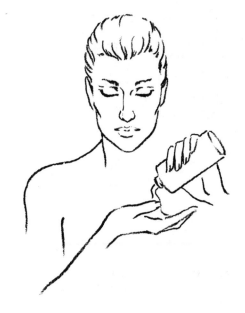

How to shampoo

• After gently combing your hair to remove tangles, wet it completely with warm water.
• Pour a little bit of shampoo in your hand (many hair stylists suggest diluting commercially prepared shampoos because they are very concentrated) and massage it into your scalp with your fingertips.
• Manipulate your scalp, using gentle circular motions, then work lather through your hair.
• Rinse hair thoroughly under water, with your head lowered, then raised, running your fingers

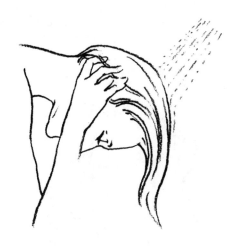

through it. When you think all shampoo is out, rinse for a few seconds longer. If you shampoo daily, you probably will not require a second lathering.
• Apply conditioner now if you need it. Pour a small amount into your hand, rub your hands together and run them through the ends of your hair, starting about two inches from the scalp.

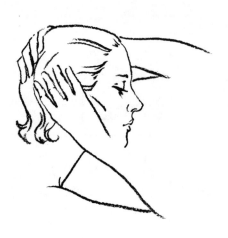

• Comb wet hair carefully, from the ends to the roots, then blot again with a dry towel.

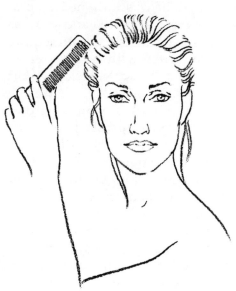

• Rinse hair thoroughly with warm water, then with cool water—a hair stylist's trick to add shine.
• Blot hair gently with a towel, then wrap the towel around your head turban-style to absorb water.

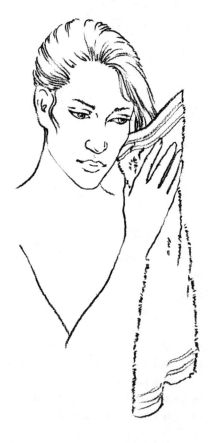

Selecting your shampoo

The ideal shampoo removes oil, scales, dirt, and dust in a gentle, nonirritating way, leaving your hair soft, shiny, and pleasant-smelling. And the best way to find it, say the experts, is by experimenting: trial and error. "But don't look for one shampoo that does everything," says Leland Hirsch. "The same shampoo can't effectively cleanse, condition, add body, and whatever else, all at the same time." He advises choosing the product that fills your needs at the time, and if you don't know what you need, speak to your hair stylist for guidance. "Also, the fewer ingredients the product contains, the more effective I find it is," he adds. Among his recommendations are shampoos that contain mild moisturizers for hair that's dry and brittle—look for the words "emollients," "oils," and "E.F.A." (essential fatty acids) at the end of the list of ingredients. This means that there are few in the formula and the shampoo will still cleanse efficiently. Hair that is porous, that stretches, needs ingredients that make it tighter and more compact. Shampoos with a lower pH and those that contain protein or nucleic acid help build up hair temporarily. Another reason for switching shampoos is to avoid the consistent action of any one ingredient. After a time, he explains, a strong protein shampoo will be too drying, while a moisturizing formulation will be too softening. The action of the two will be balanced if you alternate between them.

How important is pH?

A product's pH tells you its degree of acidity or alkalinity. Explains Dr. Norman Orentreich, a specialist in hair as well as skin, "From a health point of view, the pH balance of a shampoo is not especially important; pH balance only matters from a cosmetic point of view because keratin has certain physical characteristics in an acid pH that it doesn't in an alkaline pH." This means that your hair, which is primarily composed of keratin, will feel different after an alkaline shampoo than it will after a more acidic one.

A neutral or balanced pH shampoo seems to suit most people—and you'll find most shampoos in this category, whether it's indicated or not. A *very high* pH shampoo is harsh, while a *very low* pH shampoo can't cleanse properly. Condi-

tioners, by virtue of their function, are low pH or acidic.

CONDITIONING

"A conditioner neutralizes hair's pH after shampooing so that it feels softer and smoother, it makes it more manageable and lustrous so it looks better," states Dr. Orentreich. "It's important for the woman who shampoos often, or who has had a lot of chemical processing. It also reduces static effects." He points out too that there is no difference between an instant and a deep conditioner. "All conditioners have the same penetrating power—they are all superficial." When speaking of additives like protein, he explains that it does not nourish the hair—"the only way that protein does nourish hair is if it's eaten!" Nor does it heal hair, but it is "modestly beneficial cosmetically" because it makes hair feel better, building it up to some degree, even though the effects are only temporary. And the best way to find the right conditioner for your hair is again by trial and error.

But not all hair needs conditioning all of the time or even some of the time. Remember, hair on the dry side has the best body. And while damaged hair can certainly be helped by conditioning, it won't be healed; the damage will remain until it grows out and is cut off.

If you do use a conditioner, think of it as a finish, as Michael Mazzei does. Don't saturate your hair with a heavy formulation. Use just a little and on hair ends only. Conditioners—and this term includes cream rinses as well since they are often exactly the same—should be thoroughly rinsed out, otherwise they can leave a dulling film over your hair that will drag it down.

SETTING LOTIONS AND HAIRSPRAYS

Both setting lotions and hairsprays are body-boosters. They coat the hair. But while hair looks and feels thicker, it can become dirtier faster. Select a lightweight setting lotion, a nonalcohol type if your hair is dry, and if your hair needs more hold, try a controlling gel that has a thicker consistency than a setting lotion. A hairspray holds hair with a fixative so that it stays groomed. Always select one with soft staying-power. You never want a rigid or rock-hard look.

NURTURING ABUSED HAIR BACK TO HEALTH

When your hair is badly damaged, it needs help fast, with techniques that correct the damage and those that will prevent further damage. To get back the bounce, the glow, the life, Stephen Jacobs recommends taking these five early steps:

1. Examine your life-style, your diet. If they are not healthy, you can't expect the hair growing out of your scalp to be.
2. Speak to your stylist about a new cut that's wash-and-wear, so you don't have to rely on appliances and equipment to look good.
3. Stay away from blow-dryers and heated appliances, if possible, because heat is damaging to already damaged hair. Avoid hairsprays and setting lotions that coat and stiffen hair.
4. Condition your hair every time you shampoo—use a richer conditioner once a week.
5. Hold a moratorium on coloring your hair if the coloring method you use is causing damage. Consult with your colorist about a change in process.

A WORD OF CAUTION ABOUT THE SUN

The sun dries out hair the same way it does skin—since both are composed of basically the same substance. It renders hair dry, dull, and brittle, often to the point where it simply snaps off. It changes hair color, particularly when hair is color treated. In the sun, protect your hair with a scarf or hat. When that's not possible, use a hairspray with sunscreen. If hair is dried from sunbathing, shampoo with a mild formulation, then condition.

BLOW-DRYING IN BODY

By blow-drying your hair with your head lowered, you can give it more volume and fullness—especially if you dry the roots first, fluffing and lifting your hair with your fingers or with a wide-bristle brush in the direction opposite to the one you want the hair eventually to go. You have to keep the dryer continually moving over the area you are working,

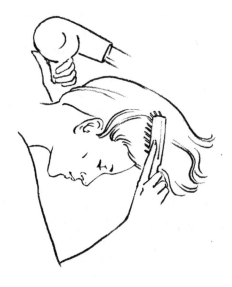

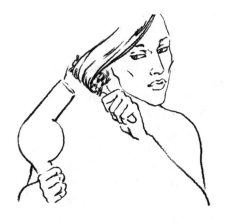

You can control voluminous hair by blow-drying it in the direction it grows, both from underneath hair and on top of it. Keep air-velocity high so that hair dries quickly, then style with a wide, round brush for looser curl. You can also wind wet

holding it about six inches from your hair. To keep the heat from becoming too concentrated, use a wide-nozzle dryer, or a dryer plus diffuser if hair is curly. Dry your hair first with lowered head, then with your head straight. Direct the flow of air from underneath until your hair is 50 percent to 75 percent dry before you use a brush to style it. If you are not handy, consider a dryer with a brush attachment.

When buying a blow-dryer, select the lightest model that has different settings in heat and air-flow control—not every head needs the same drying power. The stronger the setting, the hotter the air and the more powerful the flow of air—good for thicker, straighter hair or curly hair you want to straighten slightly. A midrange setting should be sufficient for finer hair and curlier looks, while a low setting is good for the finest, most delicate hair. To offset dryness, use one of the spray conditioners formulated for use with heated appliances.

hair on large rollers to smooth and shape it.

SEVEN FAST WAYS FOR FULLER HAIR

1. Shampoo often; hair is thickest when it's clean.
2. Comb wet hair through with setting lotion before you blow it dry or set it.
3. Blow-dry hair with head lowered, finger-combing all hair forward.
4. Have a body wave for fullness and bounce without curl.
5. Cut your hair in soft layers to release its weight. If it's very thin, have it blunt-cut all one length but no longer than your chin; too long, and it will separate and look wispy.

6. Set your hair with rollers rather than pin curls for fuller curls.

7. Backcomb your hair lightly to build it up. But realize that there's a fine line between full and too full. Stephen Jacobs observes, "Too much volume and a woman looks like she's trying too hard!"

DANDRUFF

Dandruff means scale that can be caused by many conditions, explains Dr. Orentreich. It represents several things: scaling at the surface of the scalp from the skin itself, scales from the cuticle and the sheath of the hair, sweat, dirt from the outside, and oil. It's not age-related nor does it necessarily increase or decrease through the years. But it may become more noticeable as you grow older, since the oil that would normally hold it onto the scalp diminishes around menopause. The loose scales then flake off and fall. "The most sophisticated way of correcting dandruff is to shampoo often—every day—with a gentle shampoo that you like," advises Dr. Orentreich. "This usually solves most problems." If it does not solve yours, he then suggests switching to a dandruff shampoo—one that contains tar, sulfur, selenium, or zinc omadine. "But it's a case of trial and error until you find the product that works best for you," he says. "Some antidandruff ingredients are helpful to dandruff of certain causes and aggravating to others." If nothing seems to solve the problem, it's time to consult a physician and probably a dermatologist, who can recognize the variety of your condition, who will prescribe the appropriate anti-dandruff and, possibly, antiinflammatory solution.

HAIR LOSS

Hair does not grow at a constant rate, nor does it grow indefinitely. It grows faster in summer than in winter and it grows in cycles. The growth phase of scalp hair, which generally lasts for between two and six years, is followed by a resting phase that lasts for a few months. The old resting hair falls out and a new growing hair replaces it. At any one time, 85 to 90 percent of scalp hair is in the growing phase, while 10 to 15 percent is in the resting phase; this results in a natural shedding of between 50 and 150 hairs a day in a randomly distributed pattern throughout your scalp. As the growing phase shortens through the years the ultimate length of hair shortens. And since hair growth is controlled by the hormones, as the hormone ratio changes estrogen levels are no longer high enough to counteract the inhibiting effects of androgens on hair growth. Some women lose a significant amount of hair in the years after menopause—hair that does not grow back.

If your hair falls out in excess of 50 to 150 per day or in patches, you should see a dermatologist, one who specializes in hair, to determine why. There can be many causes. Alopecia areata, for example, in which a patch of hair falls out, may be caused by a special type of self-allergy to your own hair follicles. Dr.

Orentreich explains that it may actually improve without any treatment, because allergies clear up by themselves, but it may also, if not treated, go on to quite extensive and possibly permanent hair loss.

Noticeable and dramatic hair fallout can be successfully treated, says Dr. Orentreich, who outlines the course of action he takes when this occurs. During the first visit he examines the scalp and hair in order to make a clinical diagnosis from among the twenty-five or so different causes for scalp hair loss. He draws blood for a battery of tests measuring the chemicals within it affecting hair growth. He then prescribes conservative treatment based on his clinical diagnosis. When the test results are available, he will adjust the previous therapy if necessary to correct any imbalances or abnormalities the blood tests revealed. Hormonal rebalancing may take a year or two.

Sometimes, though, irreversible hair loss has been severe enough to warrant transplanting. "I do one woman for every ten men," he says. Transplants involve taking a graft of hair follicles—about eight to fifteen—from a donor site and planting it into the bald area. This donor site is usually at the lower back of the scalp where there is no thinning. These grafts then continue to grow hair just as well as they did in their original sites; hair growth starts within three months. About fifty to sixty grafts can be done in one visit—the number of visits required depends upon the size of the bald area.

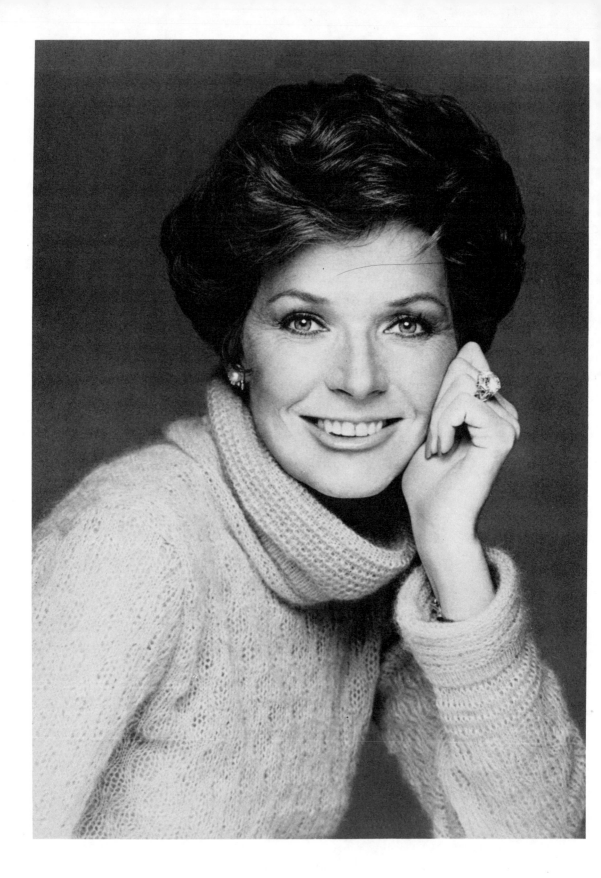

Polly Bergen

Actress, businesswoman

I think most women look better when they get older. Pretty girls are a dime a dozen—and even when I was one, I didn't find them particularly appealing. I always wanted to have character—to be a little offbeat-looking, which I find more interesting. It takes a certain amount of living to know how to really enjoy life and take care of yourself. For me, there's a sureness, an awareness, about myself now—I see it in my friends, too—a certain attitude about life that's stylish and attractive, that very few young girls have.

Socially, I think it's difficult for women now, both older and younger ones. I am seeing more and more younger men with older women. By and large, it's come out of the women's movement—women in their thirties have gone through a metamorphosis and changed tremendously, but men of the same age have not. They see us the way we used to be—as clay to work with. So they feel more comfortable with an eighteen-year-old who hasn't found herself yet and needs a father. Younger men, however, seem to be caught up in this change in women. They're fascinated by an older woman, her experience and know-how, and are less apt to be interested in an unformed young girl.

I've always had an enormous ego about my body—much more than my face—and have always cared for it. In fact, a great body was always my little secret. I never dressed in a way that showed it off, so that when summer came, people would be stunned when they saw me in a bikini. For twenty years I exercised three times a week—I was in California. But now I'm back in New York and haven't been exercising regularly—although I do bicycle everywhere—I feel my body going. It's the kind of thing you don't see as much as you feel. Actually, I can still put on a bikini and look good, but I've got to get back to exercising, and with someone who comes to my house. My schedule is hectic, plus I have no willpower and need to know I can't get out of it.

I cleanse my face with soap and water. When I had my cosmetics line, I included a soap because I knew there were a million and one women out there who did not feel clean without it. I remove my makeup with cleanser, lather with soap, rinse with water, followed by a mild, antidrying freshener. I can't leave the house without moisturizer. I would literally be in physical pain because my skin is so dry, it almost cracks. And I'm a big fan of the Buf-Puf—my skin would be in better shape if I used it more often.

When skin gets looser and looser, there's no doubt that plastic surgery is the answer. I believe in it for all the right reasons. A woman who uses it for the wrong ones is in for disappointment. It should make you look like you've had a terrific rest. You may pick up a few years on the aging cycle too, but if you expect to turn into Liz Taylor at twenty-five, you're in for a big letdown.

My makeup has changed a lot. I think that as you get older you should wear less. Like most women, I actually look ten years younger without makeup, but rarely go without it because I have thin Irish skin—it has a lot of red in it, is sensitive and blotches easily. I correct my skin tone with foundation but use less and less color on my face, except for my cheeks, which I color more and more. While bright lipsticks give a lift, I tend to wear natural shades because they have no blue in them—I find blue looks better on the young. My eye makeup is always neutral—browns, grays, earth tones. My attitude is that if you can see the makeup, you've made a mistake. I use shadow as a spotlight and do "plastic surgery" with dark matte colors: I draw in my own crease to offset the fatty area above the eye that starts to drop, and use shadow under my lower lashes, too.

My hair like the rest of me is dry, and condition is my big problem. I've always worn it short. My hairstyle calls for backcombing, which is hard on it. So is a curling iron—which has to be used to control my hair when I'm filming so that it looks the same from day to day. It needs frequent conditioning treatments, but they make it soft as duckfeathers, so I'm always stuck between wanting a treatment and hating to have one. My hair, though, has changed enormously—it used to be much thicker. I always had so much hair that it had to be professionally thinned every three weeks—now I want all the hair that was thinned out, back! I've been gray since my twenties but use color. I switched from dye, which made my hair too red, to a temporary rinse—it washes out, with the result that my hair changes color from the beginning of the week to the end.

When I think of the money women have spent on diets, I want to shake them. I am violently opposed to nut diets. Any new diet makes me angry. I have friends who have lost a thousand pounds. It's an outrage to the body— all that skin has to go somewhere, so it hangs. Dieting can only be done by changing your attitude, and a diet you can't live with for the rest of your life is impractical, a fad. I eat a gigantic breakfast—juice, two eggs, four slices of bacon, two of toast, coffee, is not uncommon—a medium lunch, and a light dinner. Often, I'll have a late brunch, then dinner, and grab an apple or grapefruit at four or five o'clock. I'm not crazy about meat, or sweets, but bread with butter or cream cheese is my downfall. The one diet I might go on is a bread diet. I love eggs and have no problem with cholesterol, or blood pressure. I am a heavy smoker—it's not something I'm proud of—but I have no intention of giving it up.

I'm a classic do-as-I-say, not-as-I-do person. Knowing what I know, being busy, impatient, and nonnarcissistic, if I can't do something quickly and easily, I just won't do it. Because sometimes it's a choice between taking care of Polly and getting involved in the activities that keep me young. I'm acting again now. I began as a singer, then became an actress. Although I've been involved in every aspect of show business, I've always been interested in business and *went into it full time in the late 1960s. I was entering my late thirties and ran a cosmetics company almost single-handedly for ten years. I do charity work. I'm writing my fourth book. I'm on the board of several companies and lecture about self-help. In addition, I have some special marketing projects, and I'm producing an idea I recently sold to Warner Bros.*

I feel I've improved with age. I know who I am, and out of that comes everything: dealing with strengths and handicaps, knowing how to dress and make up, being comfortable in my skin.

Part IV

Your Body After 40

Chapter 11

Diet: Losing Weight Without Losing Your Looks

If you think you're gaining weight more easily now, you're right—but it's probably due less to age than to inactivity. "When you become less active, you need fewer calories," explains Dr. Jaime Rozovski, assistant professor of public health at the Institute of Human Nutrition, College of Physicians and Surgeons, Columbia University. "And if you're eating the same amount as you always did, you'll gain weight." Add this to the fact that with age your basal metabolism lowers—your body is using fewer calories to perform vital functions. If you don't eat less or step up your activity, you'll put on weight. It's estimated that after the age of twenty-five the average American gains about a pound a year.

But even if you weigh the same as you did at twenty-five, body composition changes throughout the years; unless you've exercised faithfully, you're fatter now: the percentage of fat in the body increases while muscle mass decreases. And you require fewer calories to maintain this fat tissue since it uses less energy than muscle tissue. To reestablish the necessary balance, you must eat less to lose fat, and exercise more to gain muscle. Both are important,

because diet alone can lead to a loss of lean tissue along with fat, which would be counterproductive. Remember—diet slims, but exercise reshapes (more about it in the next chapter).

Now, too, you have to be even more careful about how you lose weight—a too-rapid weight loss or a plan without the proper nutrients is devastating to your system, thus your looks. Your skin has lost the resiliency that let it bounce back into shape when you were a teen-ager. It can no longer compensate for mistakes. You have to nurture it, with the right nourishment, the right calories. Because not all calories are alike; some provide more nutrients than others.

ALL CALORIES ARE NOT CREATED EQUAL

A calorie is a unit of energy. All of the foods we eat—proteins, fats, and carbohydrates—are metabolized to produce energy, measured in calories. Body processes burn up a certain amount, and physical activity burns up more. You lose weight when you take in fewer calories than you use up. One pound of body fat equals 3,500 calories—thus, to lose a pound, you have to cut your calorie intake by 3,500 or expend that amount in physical exertion.

The body, however, cannot differentiate between calories from one source over another, in terms of gaining weight. Eat more calories than you use up and you'll put on pounds—3,500 calories, whether they be from chocolate or from carrots, still add up to one pound. You usually gain weight from the chocolate because you're likely to eat more of it before you feel full, since more calories are packed into a smaller amount. With carrots you're satisfied eating less because the calories are contained in a larger quantity.

It's only in terms of nutrition that the body knows the difference between calories. Carrots provide more nutrients than chocolate, and when you get those that you need, you look better, stay healthier.

LOSING WEIGHT WITHOUT LOSING YOUR LOOKS

Basically, you must learn how to get the most nutrients from the smallest number of calories. "Your diet has to be balanced and varied," says Dr. Rozovski. "Not all nutrients are present in one single food, so it's important to eat a variety of foods to make sure you get what you need." Fad diets are hard to adhere to for more than a week or two because they don't offer enough variety. They're also unhealthy because they're not balanced, and so deprive your system of the tools it needs long term to keep your body running efficiently. You risk shedding pounds too quickly, before your skin can adjust accordingly, and often the loss is not fat at all, but water. While the initial water loss is not great on a balanced diet, you'll be losing what you need to lose. "The body is an intelligent organism," says our expert, "it tries to preserve the tissues it thinks essential. Muscles are more important than fat, so you lose fat first. Then, if you run out of fat and your diet doesn't contain enough protein as well as calories, you'll lose muscle." But, your muscle mass is on the decline after forty—you can't afford to sacrifice any of it for the sake of a fast few pounds.

THE IMPORTANCE OF WEIGHT

Obesity is linked with disease—diabetes, heart disease, high blood pressure—while maintenance of a leaner silhouette goes along with good health and a long life. Just how lean you should be, however, is currently under investigation. Some statistics show that heavier people—those who weigh more than the "ideal" weight for their frame and height—who don't have any of the complicated diseases, live longer than slimmer people. Dr. Rozovski stresses that ideal weight differs even for people of the same height and frame—that the proportion of fat in the body has to be considered.

The average percentage for women over forty is above 30 percent; ideally, it should be much lower, closer to 20 percent. You can take a test to determine how much fat you carry, but an objective look in a full-length mirror can probably tell you all you want to know.

Aerobics expert Dr. Kenneth H. Cooper developed this "ideal" weight formula for the Hoffmann-LaRoche Fitness III Program, which can give you a basic guideline:

Height in inches times 3.5 minus 108 equals weight (add 10 percent if your wrist measurement is more than 6.5 inches).

Once you know what your weight should roughly be, calculate the number of calories you'll need to maintain it by multiplying by:

14, if you're not very active
15, if you're moderately active
16, if you're very active

Then adjust your eating accordingly. So, if you're moderately active and want to stay at 123 pounds, you should consume (15 times 123) 1,845 calories daily. If you want to eat more, you have to raise your activity level or you'll gain weight.

YOUR NUTRITIONAL NEEDS

The diet most of us eat may be hazardous to our health—the death rate for diet-related disease has increased alarmingly. That's why the new dietary guidelines established by the government make sense, especially after forty, when there are changes in body composition, metabolic rate, and organ systems. These guidelines call for the following: that you maintain your ideal weight; eat a variety of foods; avoid too much fat, saturated fat, and cholesterol; eat more fruits, vegetables, and whole grains for their complex carbohydrates and fiber; and cut down on sugar and salt and alcoholic beverages. However, even the experts do not agree about nutrition—as you might have already guessed from the proliferation of books on diet.

The role of supplemental vitamins in the diet is another unresolved issue. "If you're eating a balanced and varied diet, I don't advocate supplements," states Dr. Rozovski, "because there's no danger of a vitamin deficiency. However, if you're taking a supplement very high in the fat-soluble vitamins—A, D, E, and K—you may want to reconsider it because these vitamins, especially A and D, can be toxic in large doses." Generally, a reduced-calorie diet (under 1,200 calories, according to some experts, and 1,500 calories according to others) does not supply all of the recommended and needed nutrients—particularly iron, which is important in adequate amounts and, especially if you are premenopausal, may be in short supply since iron in the blood is low every month—so a multivitamin preparation, or one "plus iron," is a good idea. Remember, vitamins should always be taken on a full stomach.

DIET TIPS TO KEEP YOU ON TARGET

Whether you want to lose 2 pounds or 20, these tips should keep you on the right track:

• Try not to weigh yourself more than once a week. That's when you'll see a gratifying weight loss.

• The food you serve should please the eye as well as the palate. Present it invitingly.

• Always sit down at the table to eat; never eat when you're standing.

• Don't keep second helpings at the table. Once you've served yourself, put leftovers away.

• Only eat when you're hungry; stop eating when you're full.

• From time to time save some of your calories for foods you crave—which may not be part of your diet. It's important that you do not feel deprived.

• Don't be discouraged by an occasional overindulgence—even if you haven't compensated for it calorically. Simply cut back on your next meal and continue with your diet.

• Drink a glass of vegetable juice or snack on a low-calorie fruit or vegetable before a meal, to cut your appetite.

• Drink water before and during meals to fill you as well.

• "Decalorize" your menus by cutting down on fats—substitute skim milk for whole milk, try cooking sauces without butter or oil, broil fish with a touch of wine instead of butter.

• Reduce the amount of salt you use. It holds in water and hides weight loss.

• Nibbling has no place in a weight-loss plan—take up knitting or crocheting or any hobby that will keep your hands busy and out of the cookie jar.

• Don't read or watch television while you eat—you'll associate food with these activities. Concentrate on your meal, and only your meal, when your're at the table.

• Shop for groceries after you've eaten. Food "mistakes" often occur on an empty stomach.

• If you're still hungry after your first serving, try to wait twenty minutes before giving yourself seconds. It takes that amount of time for the stomach to signal the brain that it's satiated.

• Save your calories for the time of day you need them most. Thus, if dinner is an important social event as well as a meal, juggle your calories throughout the day so you'll have enough left to enjoy yourself at night.

• Exercise gently before you eat. It can cut your hunger.

• Give yourself a diet goal—if it means taping a picture of yourself in a bikini to the refrigerator door so you'll be reminded of those 10 pounds you want to shed, do it.

AN EFFECTIVE APPROACH TO DIETING

Losing weight without losing your looks usually involves a change in food habits, certainly if you have more than a few pounds to shed. For best *long-term* results, the experts advise a plan that is sane, varied, and flexible and that will result in a weight loss of no more than 2 pounds a week. The majority of your calories should come from complex carbohydrates—fresh fruits and vegetables, whole grains. Fats should be curtailed, and protein should make up only about 20 percent of your diet.

However, when it's a matter of "only 5 pounds" and a need for fast feedback, a *short-term* diet can gratify instantly. It can also provide the incentive to change habits so that weight never again accumulates. This diet, though, involves a different set of rules: It should be *quick*—longer than a week and you'd probably be too bored to go on—*inflexible*, to eliminate choice, thus preoccupation with menu, and *simple*, to keep you out of the kitchen. Try it for no more than seven days at a time, supplemented with a multivitamin–mineral preparation. Total calorie count, approximately 1,000.

THE FAST FEEDBACK SEVEN-DAY DIET

Day 1:

BREAKFAST

> 1 poached or soft-boiled egg
> 1 slice whole wheat toast with 1 tsp. margarine

MIDMORNING SNACK

> Stays the same every day: select 1:
> 1 apricot, 1 small apple or pear, ½ orange, ½ cup pineapple, wedge of melon or grapefruit, or a handful of grapes

LUNCH

> 1½ cups fruit salad with ½ cup low-fat cottage cheese, sprinkled with 1 tbsp. chopped walnuts
> 2 slices crisp bread

MIDAFTERNOON SNACK

> Stays the same every day: 6 oz. vegetable juice or a selection of raw vegetables: carrots, cucumbers, celery, and radishes

DINNER

Tossed green salad with 1 tbsp. low-calorie dressing
Broiled scallops on a skewer: ¼ pound scallops threaded on a skewer
   with a quartered onion, 5 cherry tomatoes, red or green peppers,
   and brushed with a mixture of soy sauce, lemon juice, and grated
   ginger
½ cup brown rice
½ cup steamed green beans
½ cup fresh pineapple

Day 2:

BREAKFAST

1 cup bran cereal
5 sliced strawberries
¾ cup low-fat or skim milk

MIDMORNING SNACK

LUNCH

¼ pound small cooked shrimp on a bed of mixed greens with sliced
   tomatoes, carrots, and raw broccoli with 1 tbsp. low-calorie dressing or cocktail sauce—a mix of catsup and horseradish
1 slice Melba toast

MIDAFTERNOON SNACK

DINNER

Salad of tomato and lemon slices with basil, 1 tbsp. low-calorie dressing
Broiled filet of flounder: small filet topped with a mixture of 1 tbsp.
   low-calorie mayonnaise, ½ tsp. Dijon mustard, and chopped fresh
   parsley, then broiled
½ cup steamed zucchini
½ baked acorn squash
Small wedge melon

Day 3:

BREAKFAST

½ orange
½ bran muffin
½ cup low-fat cottage cheese

MIDMORNING SNACK

LUNCH

Large green salad, a mix of any of the following vegetables: bean sprouts, green beans, broccoli, beets, carrots, cauliflower, cucumbers, lettuce, mushrooms, peppers, onions, radishes, zucchini and tossed with 1 tbsp. low-calorie Italian dressing, sprinkled with Parmesan cheese
2 whole wheat bread sticks

MIDAFTERNOON SNACK

DINNER

Endive and watercress salad with 1 tbsp. low-calorie dressing
Broiled skinless chicken breast—marinated in lemon-lime juice and oregano
Small baked potato
2 spears broccoli, steamed
1 small pear

Day 4:

BREAKFAST

½ grapefruit
1 slice whole wheat toast with 1 slice diet cheese

MIDMORNING SNACK

LUNCH

Cold pasta salad: 1 cup whole wheat pasta tossed while still warm with 2 tbsp. low-calorie Italian dressing, 1 tbsp. grated Parmesan cheese, diced pepper, tomatoes, scallions, and broccoli flowerets. Chill.

MIDAFTERNOON SNACK

DINNER

Chopped green salad with celery and carrots, 1 tbsp. low-calorie dressing
Small broiled veal chop
½ cup stewed tomatoes and herbs
1 small peach

Day 5:

BREAKFAST

> Wedge melon
> 1 slice whole wheat toast with 1 tbsp. peanut butter

MIDMORNING SNACK

LUNCH

> Curried tuna salad: 1 small can water-packed tuna, mixed with 1 tbsp. low-calorie mayonnaise, curry powder, lemon juice, ¼ cup diced apple, 1 tbsp. raisins, served on a bed of greens with carrot and celery sticks
> 1 slice crisp bread

MIDAFTERNOON SNACK

DINNER

> Tomato and onion salad with 1 tbsp. low-calorie dressing
> Eggplant marinara: 1 broiled slice of eggplant baked with tomato sauce, topped with a slice of skim-milk mozzarella and a sprinkling of Parmesan cheese
> 1 cup fruit salad

Day 6:

BREAKFAST

½ cup blueberries
1 baked egg with a sprinkling of Monterey Jack cheese
1 slice whole wheat toast

MIDMORNING SNACK

LUNCH

1 cup Manhattan clam chowder
Large mixed green salad with 1 tbsp. low-calorie dressing
1 whole wheat bread stick

MIDAFTERNOON SNACK

DINNER

Red cabbage, peppers, and carrot salad with 1 tbsp. low-calorie dressing
½ small lobster, steamed
1 small ear corn on the cob
Wedge melon

Day 7:

BREAKFAST

Yogurt shake: in a blender, mix ½ cup low-fat yogurt with ½ small banana, 1 peach, or 10 strawberries, 1 tablespoon wheat germ, ⅛ cup water, lemon juice, and cinnamon

MIDMORNING SNACK

LUNCH

Large tomato sliced and served with 2 oz. part skim-milk mozzarella topped with chopped basil and 2 tbsp. balsamic vinegar
1 whole wheat bread stick

MIDAFTERNOON SNACK

DINNER

Spinach and mushroom salad with 1 tbsp. low-calorie dressing
Filet of sole Véronique: small filet of sole oven-poached in white wine, water, and herbs, topped with 1 tbsp. toasted pine nuts and sliced green grapes
½ cup brown rice
½ cup steamed green beans
½ cup strawberries

Note: You can have unlimited amounts of coffee and tea—with skim milk and artificial sweetner. You can also have as much sparkling mineral water as you wish.

FOOD FOR THOUGHT

So both your weight and the foods you eat to arrive at that weight, count. For just as your body is changing, the way it uses and is affected by foods is changing too. The following five substances should be reconsidered, then, in the light of current medical thinking:

• *Calcium*—Include more of it in your diet. Calcium is the mineral that keeps bones strong—and while it has always been considered an important element of a growing child's diet, it's often overlooked by adults. But your need for it actually increases with age, especially after menopause, when osteoporosis, a disease that demineralizes the bones, making them fracture-prone, really becomes a problem in the body and in the mouth as well, since some studies suggest that periodontal disease may in part be due to a calcium deficiency. While the exact causes of osteoporosis are not certain, it seems to be most common among women and may be related to declining estrogen levels, long-standing calcium deficiency, a decline with age of the capacity to absorb calcium, and a diet high in protein and/or phosphorous, which prevent calcium from reaching the bones. "No treatment has been discovered that stimulates bone formation," says Dr. Rozovski, "although some reduce bone loss. Estrogen Replacement Therapy is one, but along with reduction of bone loss is the increasing danger of cancer. We recommend including at least

800 mg. of calcium a day in your diet (for people showing symptoms of periodontal disease, the amount is upped to 1,000 mg. daily), and avoiding carbonated beverages (high in phosphorus) and high-protein foods." There are many doctors, however, who feel this amount is low and who are raising the dosage to 1,500 mg. for middle-aged and elderly women. The following are good sources of calcium. They are listed with a milligram count per serving size:

skim milk powder, ¼ cup, 400 mg.
collard leaves, 1 cup cooked, 360 mg.
sardines, 8 medium, 354 mg.
low-fat milk, 1 cup, 350 mg.
yogurt, 1 cup, 270 mg.
Swiss cheese, 1 oz., 260 mg.
salmon, red, 3½ oz., 259 mg.
cottage cheese, 1 cup, 230 mg.
kale, 1 cup cooked, 200 mg.
salmon, pink, 3½ oz., 196 mg.
broccoli, 1 stalk cooked, 160 mg.
oysters, 6, 156 mg.
soybeans, 1 cup cooked, 130 mg.

Calcium can also be taken in supplemental form if your diet falls short of the recommended amount, but check with your doctor first.

Vitamin D activates calcium absorption—but if you are consuming a balanced diet, it should include enough vitamin D to fill your needs. A new preparation of vitamin D may be in the works that is nontoxic and may help to decrease bone loss.

• *Cholesterol*—try to reduce your cholesterol intake. This substance is available in the diet and is also manufactured by the body from fats and carbohydrates, and its level in the blood is determined by availability from these two sources. Data indicate that a diet rich in cholesterol and saturated (animal) fat is linked with cardiovascular disease, particularly after menopause.

Cholesterol moves through the blood attached to protein carriers. These lipoproteins can be either low density (LDL) or high density (HDL). LDL cholesterol is the harmful kind, but it can be partially lowered by consuming a diet low in cholesterol and in saturated fat. This means cutting down on eggs—the highest concentrated source of cholesterol—substituting low-fat and skimmed milk products for whole milk ones, and alternating saturated fats with polyunsaturated and monounsaturated fats. Polyunsaturates (corn, safflower, and vegetable oils) appear to lower cholesterol levels, and monounsaturates (olive and peanut oil) seem not to affect cholesterol at all. Recent findings, while inconclusive, indicate a possible relationship between cancer and polyunsaturated fats, though. So while substituting polyunsaturated for saturated fat is wise, it's wiser still to reduce total fat intake, say the experts. HDL cholesterol, however, is associated with cardiovascular health. Studies suggest that it actually protects against coronary artery disease. Before menopause, women have higher levels of this kind, which could explain why the incidence

of heart disease is rare for women under fifty. But after fifty the situation changes as HDL cholesterol levels dip. This is definitely the time to closely monitor cholesterol and fat intake, and to exercise regularly and strenuously. In addition to all the other benefits exercise provides, it is believed to increase HDL cholesterol.

• *Fiber*—be sure to eat enough of it. The best sources of fiber are raw fruits and vegetables and whole grains, like whole grain breads, cereals, and pastas. Fiber aids in digestion, and there's evidence that it helps reduce the risk of cancer of the colon and other diseases, while providing valuable micro-nutrients. Other advantages of fiber-rich foods, especially important to you now when every calorie has to count, are that because of their bulk they are filling and satisfying yet not very fattening. That's why a slice or two of whole grain bread or a small bowl of whole wheat pasta with a fresh tomato or vegetable sauce can be part of your diet even when you're trying to lose weight.

• *Salt*—we consume too much of it. Salt adds flavor to foods, it's true, but it may also be true that its overconsumption increases blood pressure, heart disease, migraine headaches, and depression. Salt is found naturally in some foods—milk, meat, fish, eggs—and added to most others: almost all frozen, canned, and convenience foods. Most times you can't even taste it. If your salt intake is high, cut it to a recommended 2 grams; begin to read labels so that you know what you're eating, then try to avoid these high-salt items: salted and smoked meat or fish; peanuts and peanut butter; processed cheeses; and commercial flavorings like catsup, prepared mustard, bouillon, soy sauce, potato chips, popcorn, pretzels, and salted snacks. Offset any salt craving by adding fresh or dried herbs to add zest to your dishes, as well as spices, condiments, and vegetables like onions, peppers, and mushrooms.

• *Sugar*—you need processed and refined sugars less than ever. They supply "empty" calories—those with no nutritive value. They contribute to tooth decay, and there's some indication that the body's ability to process them in the blood decreases with age, prompting an increase in blood fat. There are also ties between sugar and diabetes, sugar and depression, and it has been suggested that there's a link between sugar and heart disease as well.

You'll find sugar in jellies, jams, candies, soft drinks, ice cream, syrups, honey, cookies, and cakes, just to name a few of the more obvious foods. In addition, sugar is contained in almost every processed food, not necessarily to sweeten, but to improve texture, retard spoilage, and add moisture. Cut down on a high sugar intake by satisfying your sweet tooth with natural sugars, those found in fresh fruits. Avoid sugared snacks and soft drinks and try new combinations of seasonings to create a sweet taste—like cinnamon, nutmeg, vanilla, and almond extracts. And always read labels on all packages of food so that you'll know what you're buying.

Chapter 12

Exercise: Toning Up the Trouble Spots

Is middle-age spread inevitable? Yes, say the experts—if you don't exercise! Because your body changes even if your weight doesn't. You become relatively fatter and less muscular with age. And that's something that the bathroom scale does not show. Diet can help you lose pounds, but only exercise can help you lose inches from those places that are bothering you now.

After forty you need an exercise program that burns off fat and builds up muscle—one that not only increases your heart's efficiency but tones up trouble spots and aids your posture, too. For there is evidence that many of the body changes associated with aging are really the result of poor fitness—and culture-related. "When a woman reaches forty and says she can't do this or that, it's not true at all," states Dr. Willibald Nagler, chairman of the department of rehabilitation medicine and physiatrist in chief at The New York Hospital–Cornell Medical Center. "She can do everything if she does it in moderation—after menopause as well. She can play tennis until her seventies."

But "Exercise is a bore," you wail. Or "I don't have time." Or "I tried it once and it didn't work." All of this might be true—for you. Especially if you're someone who does not work out or play a sport for the sheer joy of movement. So your first step is to establish a personal goal—motivation is essential. Which of the following goals will push your button and get you into motion?

WHAT EXERCISE WILL DO FOR YOU NOW

Here are eighteen good reasons—not necessarily in order of importance—to begin exercising immediately. They are all different, yet interrelated:

1. *You'll look thinner.* Muscles take up less space than fat, so a tauter body (which might actually weigh more) *seems* slimmer than a flabby one. In addition, on a diet you may lose lean body mass—just what you want to build up—as well as fat, so your body will look fatter. Only exercise builds muscle.

2. *You may not even need to lose those 5 pounds.* Why deny yourself the foods you love? Tighten those muscles and you'll look 5 pounds thinner without having to give up a single goodie.

3. *You'll lose weight faster.* Exercise increases the number of calories you expend both while you're working out and after you've finished. Diet

/151

while you exercise and you'll use even more. Contrast the following calorie expenditures, from activity, with sleeping, which burns 1.2 calories per minute:

Calories per minute

Tennis	5.2
Walking	5–7
Bicycling (5–15 mph)	5–12
Swimming	6
Jogging (12-minute mile)	10
Jumping rope	10–15

You have to cut out 3,500 calories to lose 1 pound; figure if you walk briskly just an hour a day, you'll lose close to a pound a week.

4. *You can eat more.* "Up" your activity level and you can "up" your calorie intake without gaining an ounce.

5. *You'll want to eat less.* "There's an automatic self-regulating system," says Dr. Nagler. "If you exercise regularly, you eat less."

6. *You can "spot" tone.* You can tone selectively—tighten your abdomen or thighs or buttocks, trouble spots that soften and spread with age and inactivity, unless you keep after them.

7. *Your skin color will improve.* Circulation naturally slows down with age, but exercise speeds it up, bringing a healthy rosy glow to your face. Remember, anything that benefits your overall health benefits your skin.

8. *You'll build your defenses against stress.* And therapeutically release pent-up emotion and nervous tension. So much of illness is believed to be stress-related that there is no way of measuring how much good exercise will do.

9. *You'll feel happier.* Evidence indicates that regular exercise may stimulate the secretions of "endorphins," morphine-like chemicals in the brain that fight stress and depression and promote a pleasurable sensation.

10. *You'll have more energy.* Endurance or aerobic exercise increases the flow of blood to the heart and other muscles, increasing as well the consumption and utilization of oxygen, so that you feel fitter, more energetic, stronger.

11. *You lessen the risk of heart disease.* By increasing the efficiency of the entire cardiopulmonary system, aerobics help to lessen the incidence of cardiovascular disease. They also help to reduce harmful cholesterol—the buildup of which is a problem at this age—while increasing the harmless, or HDL, cholesterol in the bloodstream.

12. *Your bones will stay stronger.* As estrogen levels change, bones become frailer, weaker, and thinner—a degenerative process known as osteoporosis. While there is no proof that bone growth and thickness can be stimulated by medication, there is evidence that they can be by exercise: when muscles repeatedly stress the bones, they strengthen them.

13. *Your posture will improve.* Strong upper-back and shoulder muscles improve and help minimize the de-

velopment of a slight humping of the upper back as you age.

14. *You'll feel more rested.* Reducing the negative effects of stress and giving the muscles the workout they want can fight insomnia, so that you'll sleep. Sleep, of course, restores muscle metabolism and is essential for total health.

15. *The risk of injury is lessened.* Exercise makes your muscles more elastic and your bones stronger, so that you're suppler and less prone to breaks and muscle tears, even if you take an unexpected fall.

16. *Your blood pressure will be lower.* Obesity and high blood pressure go together. Aerobic exercise can help you keep your weight where it should be and your blood pressure, too.

17. *You'll boost your self-confidence.* Exercise makes you look good, and looking good will help you feel good. So good, in fact, that you won't want to stop!

18. *You'll stay healthy longer.* Says Dr. Nagler: "I don't think anything beats exercise and good nutrition. They increase your defenses against illness, stress. The evidence is good that the woman who stays very active, who cares about herself and has something interesting to do, just stays healthy and young, much, much longer."

But the above goals don't have to be your goals—although some of them probably will be. Your reasons for exercising can be as simple as wanting to look terrific in a bathing suit or just loving to run around a tennis court. The only thing that matters is that you have something to strive for so you won't give up.

MAKING EVERY MOVE COUNT

Almost every move you make will benefit you in some way by burning up calories and/or maintaining muscle tone and flexibility. Right now, expend energy without even thinking about it by taking an extra step here and there: using the stairs instead of an elevator; parking at the end of the lot or getting off the bus two stops before your stop so you have to walk; dancing to the radio when you're alone at home. Remember, "Regardless of what poor shape you're in, you always have the potential to improve," emphasizes Dr. Nagler. "If you were a great tennis player but have let it go, you have a better chance of getting back into shape than someone who has never exercised. But both have potential. It's relative. The input will influence the output."

Once you've established your goal, you may find the following hints will help you keep going:

• Make an appointment. Set a regular time to exercise and try not to vary it. It will add to your sense of commitment.

• If you don't feel that you can exercise alone, find a friend with whom you can work out. You'll be able to keep each other going.

• Wear something pretty: buy an eye-catching leotard or jogging outfit.

• Start slowly, especially if you've never exercised before, and increase your time and intensity gradually. Once you get "hooked" on exercise, your body will expect it, need it, and you'll feel uneasy and uncomfortable without it.

SETTING UP AN EXERCISE PROGRAM

Your program after forty should consist of three types of exercise: *aerobic* exercises to increase the efficiency of your heart and the oxygenation of your skeletal muscles; *stretching* exercises to increase flexibility as muscles tend to shorten with age, emotional tension, prolonged sedentary work, and poor posture; and *strengthening* exercises to build and firm specific muscle groups that have become lax and weak from inactivity, resulting in telltale trouble spots. Aerobics should always be combined with stretching, preceding them to warm up muscles and following them to cool muscles down. Dr. Nagler suggests stretching for 15 minutes, working out aerobically for 45 minutes, 3 times a week (or for 30 minutes, 4 times a week), then finishing with 10 minutes of stretching. Naturally, you should work gradually up to this aerobic time—you'll learn how in Part One, which follows. Part Two of your program takes only a scant 10 to 15 minutes, to be done those days that you don't exercise aerobically. Thus, you'll be exercising daily—although your routine won't necessarily be the same every day.

The exercises that will make the most pronounced difference in the way you feel—as well as in your weight, because they are the only ones that burn away fat—will be aerobic. They involve the rhythmic contraction of the muscles that return large volumes of blood to the heart, strengthening it, as well as increased oxygen that causes changes resulting in a capacity to do more with less fatigue.

Part One: Stretching and Aerobic Exercises for Flexibility and Heart Efficiency

To prevent injury and help you exercise better aerobically, start with a series of easy stretches, known as a warm-up. New York exercise expert Lynn Edlen, whose individualized home-exercise service called Home Stretch is devised for flexibility, suggests this series, which should always be performed fluidly and slowly. She emphasizes that you should never bounce or bob when you stretch, because you risk not only tearing a muscle but actually tightening the muscle you are trying to lengthen.

The warm-up

Begin by lying flat on your back on an exercise mat or carpeted floor in a "constructive rest" position: with knees bent and together supporting each other and feet apart; arms crossed with hands at shoulders; back resting in a straight line.

1. Breathe deeply several times to release tension from the lower back.

As you exhale, concentrate on dropping your spine into the floor.

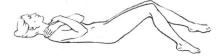

2. Stretch your legs straight out and apart with your arms over your head. Flex your hands and feet.

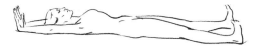

3. Stretch your opposite arm and leg away from each other, alternating sides, breathe deeply, and stretch as you exhale to lengthen your back. Do 5 times, work up to 10.

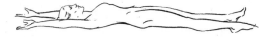

4. Leave your arms overhead and bend your knees, bringing your heels in close again. Tip your spine by pressing your lower back into the floor and slightly lifting your pelvis toward the ceiling, then releasing. Repeat, bringing your pelvis a little higher, then lower to the floor. Finally, lift your pelvis, rolling all the way up across the back of the neck, feeling a stretch in your thighs and tightening your buttocks to help lift you higher. Release slowly. It's important to sequence your spine in the proper order: Put your lower back into the floor, tip pelvis, lift through the waist, middle back, shoulder blades, and up to the back of the neck. When you lower down: Roll to shoulders, down the upper back, middle back, waist, the back of the hips, and finally the tailbone. To elongate the spine, always put

the back of waist down before lowering the buttocks.

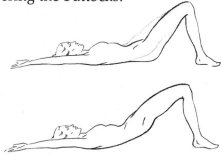

5. Put your hands behind your head, lacing your fingers together. Take a deep breath, exhale, and bring your chin to your chest and your elbows together so that you stretch the neck and back. Relax down. Do 5 times.

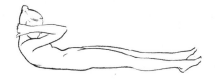

6. Bring your arms out to the sides and extend one leg. Flex your foot and, keeping your buttocks flat on the floor, raise your leg, lifting it as high as possible with the knee straight. Push through your heel to lengthen your leg, and lower your foot back to the floor. Do 5 to 10 times, then switch legs. Keep your arms relaxed.

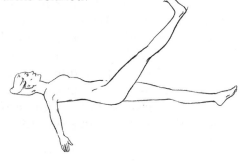

7. Bend both knees and separate your legs farther apart. Inhale, then exhale as you allow your knees to drop to one side; tighten your abdomen and let your tailbone bring you back to center. Relax and drop knees to the other side. Return to center. Exhale as you drop your legs, inhale as you bring them back to center. This is a good stretch for the lower back.

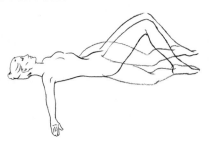

8. Pull one knee into your chest and stretch the other leg straight and off the floor, keeping your heel flexed. Take a deep breath, and as you exhale bring your knee into your chest and your forehead toward your knee. Relax everything down. Breathe in and repeat to the other side. Relax, then bring both knees into your chest with your forehead lowered. Repeat the series for a total of 5 times.

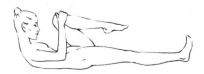

9. Taking your feet farther away so that your knees are bent just enough to keep your feet flat on the floor, stretch your arms back over your head. Tighten your abdomen and roll your chin to your chest. Float your arms forward and curl forward one vertebra at a time—keeping

your back round and shoulders relaxed—until you can drop your head to your knees and rest your hands on your ankles, leaving your head as far forward as you can. Stretch one leg out and bring it back in, then the other leg. Roll back down onto the floor. This is a moderate hamstring stretch. Do it 5 times.

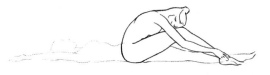

10. Sit up and cross your legs, then let your head roll: chin to chest, ear to shoulder, chin to ceiling (relaxing the back of your neck and opening your mouth slightly), then ear to the other shoulder. Do 5 in one direction, 5 in the other. When sitting upright, try to keep your torso perpendicular to the floor.

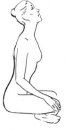

11. Put your hands on your shoulders with your elbows out to the sides, then drop elbows to ribs and bring them forward and around to the back in big circles—5 in one direction, 5 in the other.

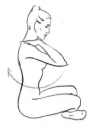

12. Bringing your hands forward, take a deep breath and slightly arch your upper back, raising your chin to the ceiling. Open your arms to the sides at shoulder height and as far behind you as you can. When you exhale, stretch your arms forward and bring your head between your upper arms as if you were going to dive, then pull your arms as far behind you as possible.

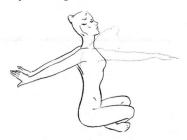

13. Put your hands back behind your head and lift your torso as tall as possible. Keeping the lift, rotate from one side to the other, 5 times to each side.

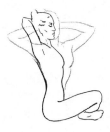

14. Rest one elbow down on the floor and, working to keep the opposite buttock on the floor, extend your other arm overhead and reach with your fingers in the direction of the stretch. This works the waist

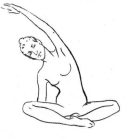

area. Alternate sides, 5 times to each side.

15. Keeping the soles of your feet together, take your feet far enough away from you so that you feel your hips relax. Allow your head to fall forward toward your feet. Concentrate on relaxing your shoulders, the back of your neck, small of your back, and front of your hips. Stay in this position for 1 minute (110 count) with your hands relaxed on your ankles. To increase the intensity of the stretch, slide your heels closer to you.

16. Lift yourself up and open your legs with knees bent. Leaning over with your hands at your ankles, stretch between your legs to loosen the thigh area. Hold the stretch for 30 seconds.

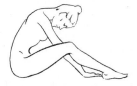

17. Sit up, tucking one leg into the center of your body and extending the other leg out as far as possible to the side with a straight knee. Keep your hands behind the back of your head and lifting your torso as tall as possible, rotate it toward your extended leg. Inhale, exhale, and drop toward the leg. Think about bringing your rib cage toward your thigh rather than your head toward your knee. This gives you a long stretch

in your back. Keep your knee relaxed and do not worry about how low your head goes. Hold 1 minute to one side, dropping your elbows and letting your upper torso become heavy, then 1 minute to the other side.

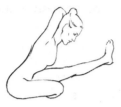

18. To do this moving stretch, extend both legs forward, flex heels, and with arms extended, reach forward as far as possible over your legs, then release the stretch and roll back to the waist; roll up again and reach, like rowing a boat. Do 5 to 10 times. (Think of flattening your navel to your spine and wrapping the sides of your rib cage toward each other so you get a scoop.)

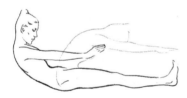

19. Cross one leg over the other at the knee, with your support on your hands. Then bring your hand over

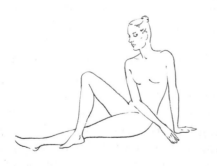

near your foot and shift into a kneeling position.

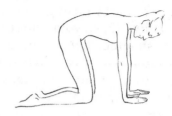

20. Do donkey kicks by rounding your back and bringing your knee toward your forehead, then stretching your leg out behind you, and lifting it while you lift your head. Work to keep your hip parallel to the floor—it's not necessary to lift your leg any higher than hip level. Concentrate on the stretch away from the body rather than the height of the leg. Inhale as you fold knee in, exhale to lift. 5 times on each knee.

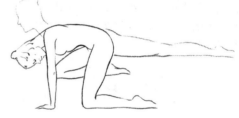

21. With your right leg outstretched, put your toe on the floor and stretch your heel down toward the floor.

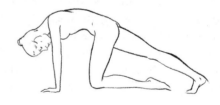

22. With the same leg, step forward and relax into your front thigh, stretching between the hips. Put your weight on your hands to return to kneeling and repeat previous exercise. Then step forward

with the left leg. Hold for 30 seconds in each position.

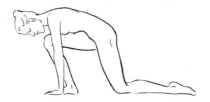

23. To get off the floor, return to kneeling, turn toes under, and press your body into an inverted V position, bringing your head as far between the arms as possible. Rise up on your toes and drop back into your heels, then tread 10 to 20 times.

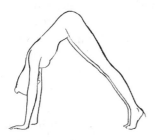

24. Come into an upright position by bending your knees slightly and walking your hands back to your feet until you are standing on both feet. Leaving knees bent, drop the top of

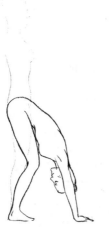

your head to the floor. Shake head "yes" and "no"; shake shoulders. With chin on your chest, tighten your buttocks and roll up, stacking one vertebra on top of the other while looking down at your feet. Relax shoulders away from ears and continue rolling up. With back straight, lift your head, and by the time you are upright, you'll find that you are standing very tall.

The aerobic workout

Your warm-up has prepared your body for the more vigorous exercise to come—the aerobic part. (If you've not exercised aerobically before, Dr. Nagler suggests checking with your doctor about your exercise tolerance. Aside from an electrocardiogram, you'll need a submaximal stress test on a treadmill. Test results can then be translated into the type of exercise best for you.)

Ease yourself into aerobics by running in place for 5 minutes or by alternating 1 block of brisk walking with 1 block of jogging for 5 minutes. Increase your time slowly—by as little as 2 minutes a week until you reach your goal of 30 minutes 4 times a week, or 45 minutes 3 times a week, the minimum amount of time necessary to maintain your cardiac reserve, according to Dr. Nagler. "If there is no sign of disease, we usually recommend exercising up to 70 percent of the heart's capacity," he explains. You can tell if you're exercising at the right intensity by taking your pulse during aerobics. After you've exercised for several months, you'll find that its resting rate will decrease as your heart becomes more efficient.

Your target training zone—the rate at which your heart should beat during aerobic exercise (70 percent of its capacity), can be established by subtracting your age from 170. Thus, if you're forty, your pulse should beat no faster than 130 beats per minute during aerobics. Check this by stopping your activity momentarily and finding your pulse with the middle fingers of your right hand on the inside of your left wrist

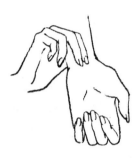

near the thumb. Count the beats for 6 seconds and add zero. If your total is higher than your target, slow down. If your target is higher than your total, build up your intensity. As exercise gets easier, you'll keep your heart rate in the training zone by building up intensity or length of time.

Aerobics are those exercises that use oxygen and involve the body's large muscle groups in rhythmic, continual action: like running in place, jogging, swimming, bicycling, jumping rope, and dancing. But while both jogging and running in place are excellent aerobic activities, they are not for everyone. As they are hard on legs, knees, and ankles, it's easy to injure yourself, especially if you have weak leg muscles. They also do little to im-

prove muscle tone in the upper body. However, they do burn up between 550 and 700 calories an hour, depending upon your speed.

Swimming, however, is perhaps the perfect endurance exercise. Says Dr. Nagler, "It affords the least danger of injury. And it's good for those with skeletal problems, because running may cause problems. Swimming also makes for very elastic muscles." When swimming, work up to at least 30 yards a minute to build your heart rate. You'll burn up between 350 and 420 calories per hour.

Consider too: aerobic dancing (classes are given throughout the country), stationary or outdoor bike riding, jumping rope—but here you have to begin extremely slowly. Rope-jumping takes time to learn. Jump for 10 or 12 turns, then recover your breath by walking around, gradually building your proficiency. Continuously jumping at a high rate of speed may take a very long time. Sports like tennis and racquetball, if they keep your heart rate in the training zone for the entire time, are good. But whatever you do, choose an activity you like, because you'll then tend to stay with it longer.

The cool-down

As you prepare to end your aerobic workout, you should gradually diminish the intensity of your activity—don't stop abruptly—then finish with the cool-down. It is designed to return your heart rate to a pre-exercise level and prevent muscle soreness and injury. Since repeated exercise tends to shorten muscles—which are then more likely to go into spasms—you have to relax and stretch your muscles to avoid any strain. An easy cool-down consists of following the exercises in your warm-up, but in reverse order. To begin, get down on the floor by simply bending your knees, relaxing down and walking your hands out 3 feet from your body, before bending your knees into a kneel; then continue with exercise 23 through exercise 1.

Part Two: Stretching and Strengthening Exercises for Posture and Problem Areas

Posture

Both posture and muscle tone count now more than ever. Your age and attitude are perhaps more apparent in the way you walk and hold yourself than in your face. Your goal is to walk taller, sit taller, keep your upper-body muscles strong to avoid slumping and developing an upper-back hump, so common with age. To improve your posture and offset problems, Dr. Nagler developed this eight-exercise plan that you can do those days you are not exercising aerobically—or daily if you have the time—coupled with several strengthening exercises to tone up jiggly areas.

Before you begin, assemble the things you'll need for this routine: a pillow, an exercise pad, a watch with a second hand, two 1-pound weights with Velcro closings (you can find these in orthopedic supply stores), and a 2½-pound can of tomatoes to use as a weight. Lie on your back with a pillow under your knees for the first 3 exercises.

1. Begin by inhaling through the nose. Blow air out slowly through pursed lips. Repeat 5 times.

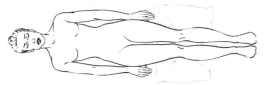

2. Roll head gently from side to side, making no effort to hold any one position. Repeat 10 times.

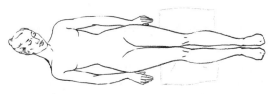

3. Shrug shoulders up toward ears, then drop them completely. Repeat 10 times.

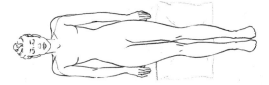

4. Standing, place palms on chest and pull shoulders down. Bring elbows to shoulder height and rotate arms 10 times clockwise, then 10 times counterclockwise.

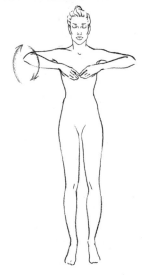

5. Lie on your back, placing hands behind neck. Bring elbows down to surface and press downward very hard. Hold 5 seconds. Relax. Repeat 10 times.

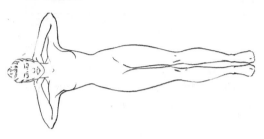

6. Go down on all fours with back straight, elbows locked. Point hands forward with palms down. Shift back and sit on your haunches, keeping hands in place but turning palms upward in shifting. Hold 5 seconds. Repeat 10 times.

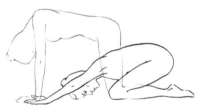

7. Sitting, take a 2½-pound weight in your right hand. Place hand over left hip, keeping arm as straight as possible. Lift the weight in an unbroken line from left hip to right

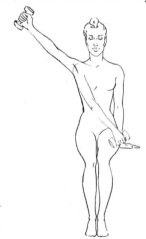

shoulder and try to reach backward. Hold 5 seconds. Repeat, alternating arms, for a total count of 5 times with each arm.

8. Lie facedown with a pillow under your stomach. Put a 1-pound weight around each elbow. Clasp hands behind your neck. Lift elbows high, hold 5 seconds. Relax 2 seconds. Repeat 10 times.

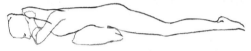

Toning up those trouble spots

Now let's zero in on those specific trouble spots—the flabby ones where inches show more than ever: the abdomen, buttocks, inner thighs, waist, and arms. They respond best to strengthening exercises, which firm specific muscle groups. Lynn Edlen suggests this set of seven exercises to tighten the areas where age makes inroads. Remember to build your repetitions gradually and to ease into a stretch without forcing or bouncing. These exercises should not hurt.

• To flatten your stomach: roll-ups. Lynn suggests lying on your back on an exercise pad with your knees bent and apart and holding a weight in front of you (a cast-iron frying pan will do nicely). Exhale as you roll up to a count of 4—flattening your navel to your spine and curling your rib cage around itself so you feel like there is a scooping motion in your stomach. Begin with 10 and increase 1 each week until you can do 25. When these get too easy, you can bring your heels closer to your buttocks, which makes them harder, or try crossing your arms over your chest, then behind your head.

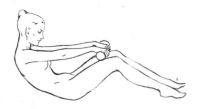

• To firm your inner thighs: Lie on your back with your arms relaxed at your sides or behind your head. Keep your knees bent and put a pillow between your legs. Squeeze for 6 seconds. Relax. Begin with 10 and work up to 25.

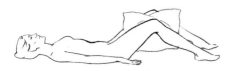

• To tighten your buttocks: kneeling on the edge of your bed, fold your arms and support your forehead on them, then straighten one leg and bring it slightly up above your hip, then down to the floor. You should feel no strain in the

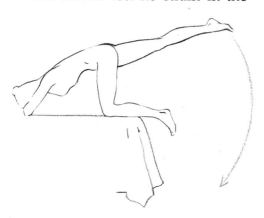

back of your waist—if you do, you are arching your back. Control your back by keeping your abdominals taut. Inhale as you raise your leg and exhale as you lower it. Begin by lifting each leg 10 times and build to 25. Increase the efficiency by adding 2½-pound weights to each ankle when you lift, and build your repetitions slowly.

• To whittle your waist: side bends. Stand with your feet slightly apart and your knees relaxed. Holding a 2½-pound weight in each hand, slide one weight down your leg and the other up your side to your armpit. Start with 10 each side (alternating sides) and build to 30. The motion is purely lateral—try not to twist.

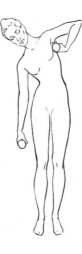

• To firm your upper arms: Stand sideways against a wall with your hand in a fist raised above your head. Bend your arm at the elbow and touch your hand to the opposite shoulder, behind your head. Exhale when you extend your arm. Your head should be straight forward, your abdomen tucked in, and your knees relaxed. Begin with 10 each side, working up to 25. When the exercise becomes too easy, hold a 1-pound weight in your hand, increasing to a 2½-pound weight when your arm gets stronger. (You can use a can of vegetables as the 1-pound weight.)

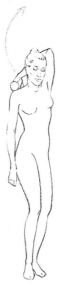

• Another exercise for upper arms is pushing against a wall—your body should be at a 45-degree an-

gle from the wall with your abdomen tucked in, buttocks tightened, and feet about 3 feet away and a foot apart with knees straight. Inhale as you try to touch your elbows to the wall and exhale as you push off and straighten your arms. Start with 10 and increase to 25.

• To tighten your outer thighs: Lie on your side with your abdomen taut and your back flush to the wall with knee of bottom leg bent, and raise your upper leg with your foot flexed. Inhale as you lift, exhale as you lower. If the exercise is difficult, push the heel of your hand into the floor. Begin with 10 each leg and increase to 25. When you get stronger, try the exercise with a 2½-pound weight around each ankle. When the exercise becomes too easy, slow it down.

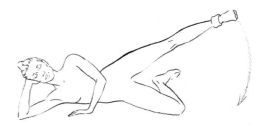

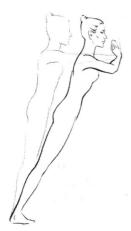

Chapter 13

Dressing Slim

Diet and exercise can shape your body, but they cannot change your basic body shape. Nor can they perfect every figure flaw. Skin that's lost its elasticity cannot get it back. The body that's never been firm and taut has a much tougher time shaping up after forty than one that's always been fit. The little problems that can come with age and that do not respond to exercise—a protruding abdomen, a thickening waist, sagging upper arms—can, however, be offset by optical illusion: controlling them with undergarments, camouflaging them with clothes, taking attention off imperfections, and drawing it to assets.

Your overall image counts most, and it begins with your attitude. Are you comfortable with yourself? "How you put yourself together— the colors, textures, accessories you use—shows others what you think of yourself, who you are," says New York image consultant Emily Cho. "After forty, you should be concerned about the message you're sending out, so that you're getting the reactions you want. You know more about what does not work for you." You tell people about yourself without even opening your mouth. And while individual tricks solve figure problems, what counts most is an interesting and finished total look. "Don't fixate on your weight and proportion; you can't change your bone structure. And it really is a bore to keep focusing on those five pounds you always want to lose. We all do it when we're twenty, but we should get over it in our thirties," advises Emily. "Work on your posture and carriage—think of a tape held between your two shoulder blades. Walk tall and keep your movements light; heavy movements are aging. Then pull your outfit together. Even if your skirt is slightly wider than you'd like for your generous hips, it's more important that the look is finished." Furthermore, there should always be a balance of what's practical—what complements your body—and what's available in the stores; you have to work within the system. After forty, you're in a state of equilibrium, of not trying too hard fashion-wise, yet keeping up with what's current. "Nothing's worse than looking like you're trying too hard," cautions Emily.

AGE AND STYLE

"I don't believe that clothes are necessarily age-related. We're more relaxed these days and not as confined to protocol," maintains Betty Halbreich, director of Solutions, the personal shopping problem-solving service at Bergdorf Goodman. So, if you've been sophisticated or sporty, frilly or even "preppie" all of your life—and you're comfortable with your personal style—you should by all means continue dressing that way. You may want to add variety to your look with different accessories, with different silhouettes, all in keeping with the overall fashion context.

"After forty, you sometimes need a whole new dimension, though," adds Betty. "If you decide you want to change what's in your closet, it could make the biggest change in your life!" For clothing is a psychological tool that you can use to boost your ego. And when you feel as if you're in a fashion rut—your children are grown and out of the house, other circumstances have changed and you want to as well—it may be the right moment to reevaluate your image. Fashion magazines can offer you an assortment of perspectives; the next step is then experimenting with clothes you may not have considered in the past, to get a feel for them. But since it's often very difficult to be objective about yourself, you may want to seek out the opinions of an expert. Large department stores frequently have personal shopping services, small boutiques sometimes specialize in putting together a look from top to toe, and free-lance image consultants can be hired on a project basis, certainly in the larger metropolitan areas. You're probably better off if you don't rely upon the advice of a friend, since it may be too subjective—someone

used to seeing you one way may not be able to imagine you differently. When Betty Halbreich solves problems, she aims to bring out a woman's best features, then lets attitude shape the rest. She suggests that a happy look is the one to strive for, whatever the fashion type; your face sets the tone, then the body follows.

But how you feel about your body also shows in your face. And according to Emily Cho, most women feel too heavy. Here is where the right clothing can create a slimmer illusion, provided it has the full support of your underwear.

UNDERWEAR—THE HIDDEN PERSUADERS

"I don't think women want to be restricted anymore. Anything too structured doesn't look right, not now—women want freedom in lingerie," Betty Halbreich opines. "The softer bra, support panty hose instead of a girdle—women over forty are buying more beautiful underthings for themselves. Years ago everything was white, or black, now it's flesh-tinted, shaded."

Certainly the right undergarments can make all the difference—in the way your body looks, in the way it moves, in the way you feel. Those with soft support slim and shape the silhouette without binding it. Anything too rigid is aging, unnatural—and uncomfortable, and discomfort makes movements heavy. The proper underthings for the body, like skin-care preparations for the face, help to compensate for figure changes in a gently persuasive way.

Buying the right bra

The experts at Vassarette cite wearing the wrong size bra as a major problem. And now the most flattering bra for your bosom is extra important, as the muscles that support the fat and soft tissue of the breasts weaken somewhat with age, yielding to the downward pull of gravity. Subtle shaping and lifting, minimizing or repositioning, makes the bustline—thus whatever you wear over it—more attractive.

Even if you have a good fitter, knowing your own bra size is important. Vassarette experts suggest the following way to measure yours: While wearing a comfortable bra—one that does not bind or cut—take your body measurement around your rib cage, along the bottom band of your bra, adding 5 inches if the number is odd (thus, if you measure 29 inches around, 29 inches plus 5 inches equals 34 inches) and 6 inches if the number is even.

Obtain your cup size by taping the fullest part of your bust, then comparing this measurement to your bra size. If it is 1 inch more than your bra size, you're an A; 2 inches—B; 3 inches—C; 4 inches—D, and 5 inches—DD.

Try on a bra by slipping the straps over your shoulders, bending from the waist so that your breasts fill the cups, then standing up and hooking the bra in the next to tightest fastener. Center your nipples straight ahead and tilted slightly up. If they droop downward, your breasts will look like they are sagging, even if they are not.

Check the lift: The fullest part of your bust should rest halfway between your shoulder and elbow. If the cup shows vertical wrinkles between the point of the breast and the spot where the strap and cup meets, you're raising your breasts too high. If there are wrinkles underneath the point, you're not being lifted high enough.

Check the fit: The bra should rest in a straight line or slightly lower in back. It should not cut into your underarms. The back should not ride up or stand away. If it does, the bra size is too big or the style wrong for your body shape. If the bra bridges in front and does not rest against the breastbone, the cup is too small. If your flesh bulges over the top or under the bottom, it does not fit. A bra that's too small will only make you look bigger—misshapen, too—by squeezing you. The bra should feel comfortable and allow you to move and breathe easily. View your back in a mirror as well, to make certain your silhouette is sleek and smooth. Under sheer or clinging clothes you may want a front-closure or pull-on style, instead of a back-closure.

Bring along the article of clothing you're buying the bra for. You want a softly rounded silhouette—never a pointed one—and you don't want your bra to look obvious. You'll probably need a variety of styles: a strapless bra for strapless tops, a contour cup for close-to-the-body sweaters and silky shirts, a sport bra for those times you're running around, and the list goes on.

But no matter what size you are, you should try for the softest cup that will best balance and proportion your body: if your bust is very large and your hips slim, you may want a minimizer; if your smaller bosom does not look as good as it could with your wider hips, you may want to increase it with a lightly padded bra. If your breasts are different sizes—a very common problem—a contour-cup bra will even them.

Here are several guidelines to help you select the proper-fitting bra for your figure:

The smaller bust:
• a *soft cup bra* may or may not have a seam and provides a natural rounded look. It's good for breasts that do not need much support.
• a *contour cup bra* has a soft fiberfill lining that gives shape and firmness, and helps fill you out. It will equalize an uneven bust.
• a *padded bra* will increase your bust by one cup size in a natural-looking way.
• an *underwire bra* adds an extra little lift—especially if it's partially padded.
The larger bust:
• an *underwire bra* gives lift—but without padding.
• a *contour cup bra* is useful if breasts are uneven.
• a *soft cup bra* should probably be seamed because it provides more structure and support than a nonseamed one. Good if breasts are a bit droopy.
• a *minimizer bra* provides maximum support while flattening and minimizing an oversized bust; usually based on lightweight wires.

Body stockings

Made of a lightweight controlling fabric, like Lycra—a mix of nylon and spandex—body stockings or suits reshape you naturally so that your figure looks tighter, sleeker. They're wonderful for slimming a heavy torso in the most comfortable way. They mold to your body like a second skin. Some are manufactured with attached panty hose, but most end at the thigh.

Those without stitched or woven panels—to flatten the abdomen, hips, or derriere—provide the lightest support. Ideally, you should purchase the least-constructed style that does what you want it to.

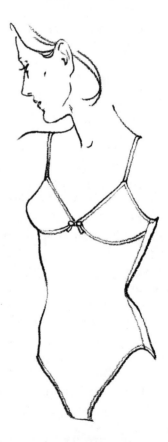

Never buy a body suit without first trying it on. Sizes differ from manufacturer to manufacturer, and it's difficult to judge the fit by simply holding the suit against you. Once you slip it on, check the following spots:

• the leg line—it should be high enough. If it coincides with the natural body line, there will be no indentation or bulge where your thigh starts.
• the crotch—it should be long enough so that you can sit comfortably.
• the waist—there should be no wrinkling here.
• the bust—the bra should offer proper support; cups should be filled with no puckering.
• the color—should not be noticeable, which is why flesh-tinted is probably best. Try your body suit on under your clothes to make certain it can't be seen.

Panty hose, etc.

If your hips, abdomen, or derriere are flabby, control-top panty hose can help firm them. Support panty hose are best for slimming heavy thighs. Regular panty hose can also help hold in the lower half of your body—but just a little. The thicker the fiber and the closer the knit, the stronger—thus more controlling—the panty hose.

Control-panel briefs, available in the same fabrics as body suits, also tighten the stomach, hips, and backside—they shouldn't cut or bind, or cause bulges at the top or bottom. While most panties can't take inches off, they can appear to

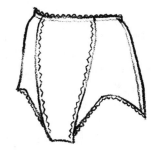

add pounds if the elastic is so tight that your flesh spills out. When you're wearing close-fitting slacks or skirts, check your back in a full-length mirror to insure that no panty lines or unsightly lumps and bumps show through.

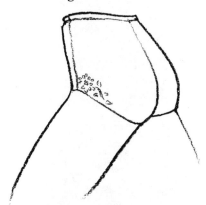

HOW TO DRESS SLIM

Longer, leaner lines and sparer shapes, supple fabrics in tones of the same shade—these are the secrets to successfully dressing slim and offsetting figure flaws at the same time. You've already established a trimmer foundation with underwear; here's how fashion—color, cut, and accessories—can also create a more lissome line:

• Begin by buying your clothing in the right size—you'll look bigger if you squeeze yourself into a smaller size. An easy line is the most flattering one.

• Silhouettes should always skim the body, never hug it. Everything should look graceful. But stay away from full dirndl skirts, puffy sleeves, voluminous shapes. Too much layering can add weight; keep layers thin so that they suggest the body underneath.

• One-color, or shades of the same color, dressing makes any body look taller and trimmer. Tone your shoes to your stockings to your

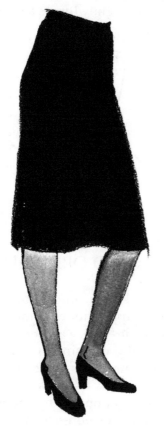

skirt or pants. Then match your shirt or sweater or jacket to the rest of your ensemble.

• Small patterns and solid colors are more slimming than large plaids and prints.

• Dark colors and cool colors—

those based on blue—tend to minimize the body more than light, bright, and warm colors—based on red and yellow. But one-color dressing, regardless of what that color is, is still more slimming than a combination of hues.

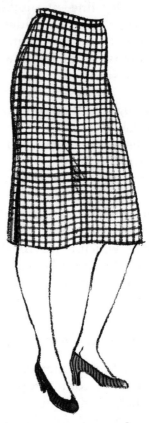

• Sling-back shoes make legs look longer and slimmer, as do open vamps and higher, more graceful heels. Avoid shoes with bows or straps—ankle straps appear to cut your leg length in half—and spike heels, too: they throw your posture out of line and into unnatural curves.

• Patterned panty hose add width to the legs. Buy solid colors or sheers, or those with a barely discernible design.

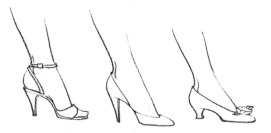

• If your midsection is thick, don't wear shoes with a lower-than-one-inch heel.
• All clothing lines should always be vertical. Avoid oversized col-

lars and wide, contrasting-color belts. Stay away from horizontal stripes or patterns.
• Bulky fabrics and accessories thicken and shorten the body. Instead of wrapping yourself up in

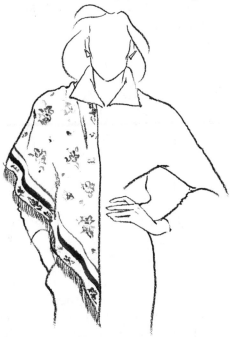

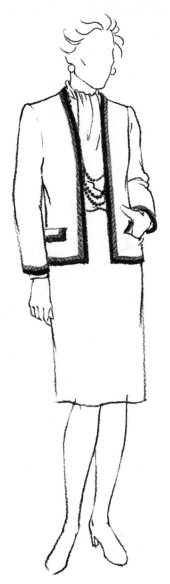

a shawl, let it dangle dramatically. Drape an oblong scarf or muffler around your neck so it hangs casually.
• Stretch a short neck with an open collar, a V- or U-neck. The

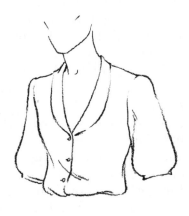

neck looks longer when a lot of skin shows, thus crew necks are more flattering and slimming than cowl necks. If your neck is too long, shorten it with a high collar, ruffles at the throat, a scarf or a turtleneck, but not one that hugs too tightly.

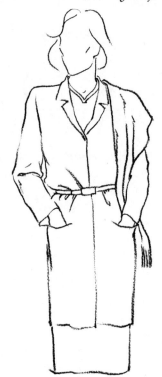

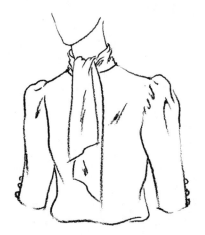

• Chokers shorten the neck while ropes of beads lengthen.

• Minimize a large bust with close-to-the-body clothes. Keep lapels narrow, shirts simple, dresses and tops draped gently. Try longer tunic tops and jackets that skim or cover your top half. Draw the eye up and away from your bustline with dramatic earrings, an eye-catching pin at your throat, a bright scarf at your neckline. Avoid details that draw attention to your bust—pockets, ruffles, elaborate yokes, horizontal necklines, double-breasted styles.

• Thin a thick waist with styles that skim or mask it—blousons, vests, overshirts, cardigans, and unfitted or semifitted jackets. Tuck shirts in, then blouse them softly. A narrow belt is fine if you match

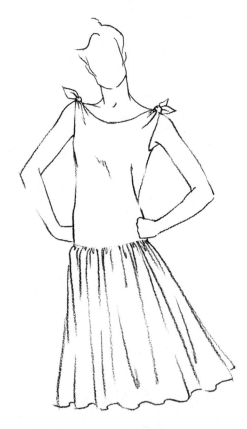

it to your ensemble. Avoid cinch belts, cummerbunds, and wide sashes. Try belting a tunic or sweater at the hip to elongate the line further.

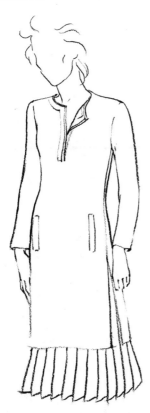

• No one will know that your abdomen protrudes if you stay away from skirts that gather at the waist and fabrics that are either bulky or cling. Opt for slim-fitting silhouettes with some give—A-line skirts, pleats that are stitched down to mid-abdomen, dresses that fall easily over your torso, that blouse gently and can be loosely sashed over sweaters and blouses. Other options are trousers with stitched down pleats, side-slash pockets, a skirt with a bit of fullness at front sides. And always stand tall.

• A high waist will look lower and the body narrower in skirts or pants with a thin waistband, or none at all. Tops should blouse gently, never hug the body, and you can let your belt—a slim one, of course—rest slightly below your waist.

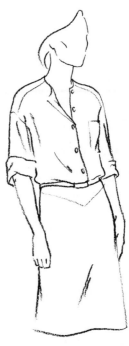

• Pleats (unless they are stitched down), gathers, horizontal patterns, and thick fabrics add inches to ample hips, as do details on pockets and loud colors. Keep the line slim—skirts that fall straight from the top of the hips, or those with a soft flare; straight-leg pants that fit impeccably (always check your rear view in a mirror), balanced with shirts and tops tucked in, then gently bloused out, as well as overshirts, vests, jackets, and sweaters that cover the fullest part of the hips. Bottoms should always be darker than tops. Pockets should be cut on the diagonal, never along the side seam. You can also draw attention away from your bottom by focusing it on your neckline, with a scarf or spot of color, or on any other area you feel is an asset.

skirts, longer cardigans, tunics, and overblouses also minimize heavy thighs without adding bulk to your overall silhouette.

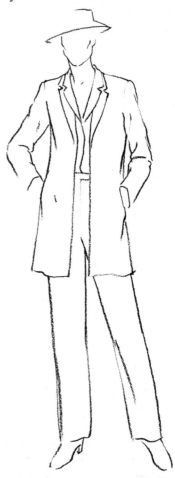

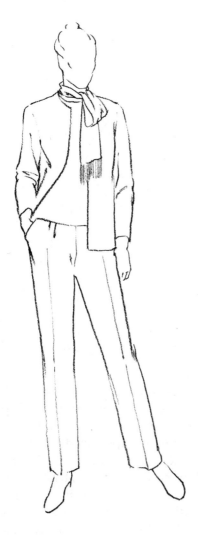

• If you're even the tiniest bit hippy, and your shoulders are narrow, never pair bottoms with skinny tops, or you'll look like a pear.
• Well-fitting trousers with straighter, slim legs, narrow-flare

• Cuffed trousers shorten and thicken the legs—you can get away with them only if you're very tall and very thin.
• Broad shoulders can be visually narrowed with raglan or drop-shoulder styles (but not if you're busty or heavy), or with sleeves set slightly inside your natural shoulder line. Strapless, halter, and V-neck tops are flattering, as are silky shirts that soften the shoulders with slight gathers.

Avoid anything that squares shoulders off—padding, cap and puff sleeves, boat necks, horizontal stripes, even turtlenecks, because you'll look broader in them.

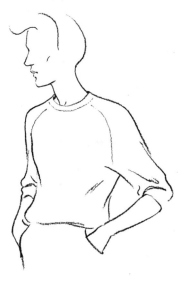

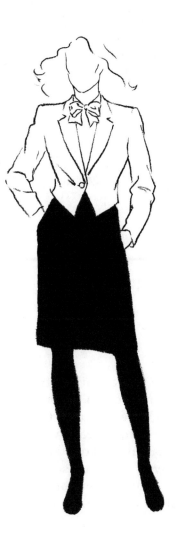

• A long torso with short legs can look more balanced by raising the waistline with a wide belt or thick sash in the same color as your trousers or skirt, then keeping bottoms narrow. Best bets: slim dirndls, straight skirts, straight-leg pants, and slightly bloused tops. Avoid low-waisted pants, belts at the hip, as well as skinny tops.

• Upper arms that are less than firm can mar an otherwise slim silhouette, so keep them covered. Soft, fluttery sleeves and long sleeves, tapered at the wrist or rolled up just beneath the elbows, provide good camouflage. Avoid sleeveless, strapless, and short-sleeve looks.

• Keep your handbag slim and in proportion to the rest of you. A big shoulder bag resting at the

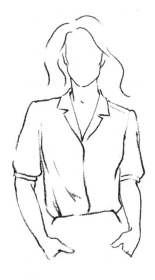

hips can emphasize them further—disastrous if yours are wide to begin with.

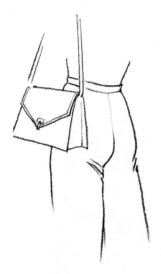

• While tall and slim is the ideal—if you're too tall, choose longer jackets, sweaters and tops to cut your length. Wear subtle colors and stay away from fussy details and oversized accessories, which only draw attention to your height.

IF YOU'RE TOO THIN . . .

Can anyone ever be too thin or too rich? Well, not too rich, perhaps—but overly thin is sometimes a problem. Fill out your figure by applying the clothing principles that slim—but apply them in reverse. Layers, thicker fabrics, and fuller lines add bulk to your body. But you should always wear your right size in order to have these tricks work; if clothes are too big, you risk looking lost in them:
  • A small or flat bosom does not

look that way when topped by ruffles, a double-breasted coat or jacket, front detailing, blousy tops, sweaters, overshirts, and undervests. Avoid anything tight or clinging, anything too bare if your chest is bony.

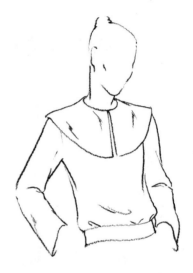

• Camouflage thin, shapeless calves with boots and trousers. When wearing skirts and dresses, keep lines simple and slim—full skirts can make your legs look thinner. Patterned and textured hose in light shades build up legs. Avoid heavy or thick-soled shoes.
• Narrow shoulders are not a problem if the rest of you is narrow as well. You can add width with gentle padding, extended shoulder lines, epaulettes, and puffed, gathered, and capped sleeves. Bandeau and V-necks, as well as small collars, seem to extend shoulders too. Steer clear of raglan sleeves and halter tops, and any style that is unnaturally big or bulky—it will make you look even narrower.

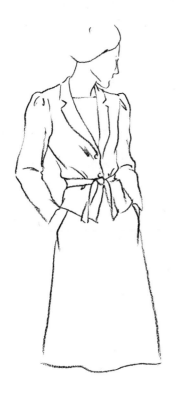

CREATING AN EFFECT WITH COLOR

"I don't think there are any 'no's' in colors. If you feel good in a color, go with it!" says Betty Halbreich. "Wearing a flattering color is the best way to get a compliment," adds Emily Cho. And whether you're dressing to whittle down your weight or add to it, the right color—one that complements your looks, and the lines and fabric of your fashions—can create any effect you want.

It's important that you feel comfortable in the colors you wear; their choice is highly individual. You may find that it's easier and more mistake-proof to work with a limited color palette than an open-ended one, building your wardrobe around three to five shades that mix and match. If they are neutrals—tones of tan and white, for example, beiges, browns, creams—you can always liven them up with a bright accent, like a touch of red. The point to remember is that colors should be balanced, just the way fabrics and styles are; they should not necessarily always match but should harmonize and interrelate. You may also find that those colors you never thought you could wear look good as long as you keep them away from your face. The dove-gray flannel suit that sparks up your salt-and-pepper hair but drains your complexion can take on a whole new appeal if you wear it with a soft rose scarf tied at the neckline.

"You tell people through color whether or not you're ready for interaction," explains Emily Cho. "Dowdy colors—muddy, murky shades—can be depressing. Change your personality by going to a color, even before you feel ready for it. It will alter the way others react to you, thus the way you feel. You're sending out a different message, so you'll get a different response."

STAYING IN THE FASHION MAINSTREAM

Fashion is continually changing, and keeping abreast of the new looks—interpreting and individualizing them so that they are becoming to you—can do more for your self-confidence and total image than simply covering up trouble spots. Wearing clothes you feel good in, that express who you are, can give you a tremendous feeling of security, of being in control. Use these pointers to stay fashion-smart:

• Watch what the women you think dress well are wearing. Analyze what works for them, and why. Ask yourself whether these touches will work for you.

• Glance through fashion magazines, but don't study them. Experiment with the ideas you find and integrate them with what you already have. A look that's too put-together is boring.

• Emily Cho suggests updating your wardrobe and your image with at least one new outfit, or portions of an outfit, each year. If you go for three years without additions and ideas, she says, you may fall so far behind fashion that you may not know where to start in order to catch up.

Chapter 14

Body Care

You've already trimmed it, toned and slimmed it visually—it's about time to pamper your body, for beauty as well as for pure sensory pleasure.

Subject to the same internal influences as your face—your health, diet, heredity—but protected by your clothing from the external abuse of ultraviolet exposure, the skin on your body probably looks less marked by time than your face. Structurally it's generally a little thicker, too, as well as drier, since it has far fewer oil glands and small hair follicles. This oil gland density does vary, however; the chest and back are oiliest, while the rest—the arms, legs, hands, and feet—are drier in different degrees. But despite its differences from facial skin, body skin still needs the same concern and care: continued protection, the right cleansing and preservation of its natural moisture. Explains dermatologist Dr. Irwin Kantor, "As you become older, skin becomes gradually drier—it loses water. The sebaceous (oil-producing) glands become less active and there's a loss of flexibility as the fragmentation of elastic tissue increases."

Dryness is hastened by low humidity. When the air is dry, it draws moisture from every source it can, including your skin, especially when its natural protection—oil—wears thin. "You have to hydrate your skin, and the best way is by sitting in water," explains Dr. Kantor. "Then, before this moisture evaporates, occlude it." This translates to plumping up outer-skin layers with water so that they are soft and smooth, then sealing in the moisture with a rich body lotion, cream, or oil.

WATER AND SKIN

Skin moisture is, purely and simply, water. Water makes up about 70 percent of the weight of your skin (and 70 percent of your body weight, too), and is the only element that can soften skin. Moisturizers do not moisturize in the true sense; they guard the moisture already present with an occlusive film.

The best type of water for bathing or showering is soft; it allows a rich lather and easy and thorough rinsing. Hard water, water with a high mineral count, deposits a thin film on the skin that can dry and irritate it. You can test to see how hard your water is by filling a jar with distilled or rainwater and one with tap water, then adding a teaspoon of shampoo to each and shaking each vigorously. If there is less lather in the tap water, the water is hard. You can soften your water with a special converting device or by adding bath salts, which increase cleansing efficiency as well.

Water temperature also aids in the cleansing process. For optimal cleansing without any shock to your system, keep your bath or shower water at between 98° and 100°F. This temperature is most soothing because it approximates that of the body. And although you may want to go a bit cooler to wake you up, or warmer to wind you down, you should avoid sudden extremes. Water that is too hot is very fatiguing, and dangerous if you have heart trouble or are overweight. It's also drying instead of moisturizing, because you lose water as your body perspires, and capillaries can dilate and rupture as the heart becomes overstimulated. Ice-cold water can also be shocking, causing the blood vessels to constrict in an attempt to save heat, so that there is less blood flowing to the heart.

But water to cleanse is only part of the total beauty picture. Water to invigorate or, conversely, to relax is equally important for your body and your mind. The first step toward transforming your bath or shower into a beauty experience is to establish the suitable ambience.

Setting the scene

Today's bathroom can look like a salon, workshop, or harem, even if yours is just a small functional room. But whatever your theme, you want the atmosphere to be as pleasant as possible, for total and absolute indulgence. To make the most of your time in and around the tub, consider the following decorating additions:

• Yards of mirrors to see yourself clearly at all angles—they will also remind you to stick to your exercises.

• Diffused lights to cut down glare and shadows.

• Bathroom carpeting or layers of rugs to pamper your feet.

• An attractive shower curtain, prints on the walls, and shelf space for pretty personal items—perfume bottles, a collection of decorative combs and brushes, bath items.

• A heated towel rack—the height of bliss—plus thick, cushiony bath towels, to warm up, then snuggle into. If this type of towel rack is not in your future, try draping your towel over the radiator.

• Baskets of herb potpourri and scented soaps to please the eye and the senses. The warm, moist air helps fragrance flower and last and last.

• Greenery for the visual pleasure and healthy note. Plants absorb stale carbon dioxide in the air and release oxygen. If you have a window and receive sunlight, add a fern—it thrives in a bright humid atmosphere—or plant pots of fragrant herbs. If your bathroom is dark, experiment with special plant-lights.

• A small tub tray to hold your beauty essentials—tweezer (tweezing is especially easy in the tub because steam opens the pores, making hairs easier to grasp), a mirror, razor, even a magazine.

• A bath pillow to provide cushioned comfort when you're leaning back. Of foam rubber or inflatable plastic, pillows are available in a variety of sizes, shapes, and colors. In a pinch try a rolled-up towel.

In-tub necessities

Consider these as necessities, as well as luxuries. They help you cleanse better, so improve your circulation and skin tone too. Your blood flow is slower in your body than in your face—that's why a facial wound heals faster, explains Dr. Kantor—slower still as the years go by, so you really want to try to get it going.

• Sponges. They can be natural or synthetic; their fineness depends upon your skin's sensitivity: the more sensitive your skin, the finer the sponge.

• Washcloths. Usually of terry, they help you cleanse even hard-to-reach and sensitive areas. Good for all skin types.

• Loofahs. Composed of the dried seed of a tropical gourd, a loofah, because of its abrasive surface, is ideal for scrubbing away dry, flaky skin on the legs and upper arms especially, as they become scaly and rough. They have few oil glands, and the skin has a tendency to trap fine hairs. A body sponge with an abrasive surface acts in the same way as a loofah.

• Pumice stones. These small pieces of volcanic rock smooth away rough spots when dampened and rubbed gently over them. Body skin varies in cell-layer depth—the soles are thickest and prone to calluses that benefit from a daily pumicing.

• Brushes. Available with soft, medium, or stiff bristles to buff skin and stimulate circulation. One with a long handle to reach down your back is wonderfully handy.

• Bath mitts. These slip over your hand and perform the same function as a loofah. They can be made of terry, hemp, or horsehair.

For your bathing pleasure

What you get out of the tub also depends on what you put in it, and these can make the results predictably pleasant:

• Soaps: Soap, say the experts, is the most efficient cleanser, but it doesn't please all of the people all of the time! States Dr. Kantor, "I'm a firm believer in soap—and for all skin types. Of course, if your skin is sensitive and dry and soap irritates it, use something else. Select a neutral or nonsoap, like Dove or Neutrogena." True, all soaps are not alike, because mixed into the basic recipe of natural fats and oils plus alkali are often other ingredients—to tint, scent, or moisturize—but they can irritate, too. Match your soap to your skin type and skin needs. Here's a rundown to show you what you can choose from:

Castile soaps—the best are made from olive oil; vegetable oil does not provide as high a quality.
Cream soaps—emollients and moisturizers are blended into the basic soap recipe for added lubricating action.

Deodorant soaps—antibacterial agents are added to reduce odor-causing bacteria. These soaps are often too strong for dry and sensitive skin. They should not be used on the face.

Detergent soaps—these are not really soaps in the true sense. They are synthetics formulated of mild detergents and emollients. They foam well in hard water and can usually be tolerated by dry and sensitive skins.

Floating soaps—air is mixed in so that these soaps float. They have a high moisture content and lather well.

Handmade soaps—made by hand, they are high in quality, low in alkali and moisture. Expensive.

Milled soaps—mass-produced soaps of good quality. They are usually a mix of color, perfume, and soap flakes.

Oatmeal soaps—oatmeal is added for texture; it acts as an abrasive, smoothing dry, flaky skin. Good for oilier skin.

Superfatted soaps—contain extra fat or oil. Recommended for dry skin.

Transparent or glycerin soaps—low in alkali, they leave skin soft and smooth; usually lather poorly.

• Gels: these gentle, soap-free cleansers provide lots of lather. Use one in the same family as your perfume to provide a lasting fragrance base.

• Bath oils: lubricants that put the lid on moisture. Add them to your bath water after you've soaked for several minutes, because they lock moisture into the skin but prevent it from entering dry skin.

Smooth them over wet skin at the end of your bath or shower.

• Beads and crystals: these do not cleanse, but they do soften the water, adding fragrance and color to give your spirits a lift. Those with a high alkali content, however, may be irritating to sensitive skin.

• Bath milks: provide quick, fragranced foam; contain dry or liquid milk products to soften skin and moisturize it.

After the bath is over

Both heat and water soften your skin, opening its pores and making it ultrareceptive to products that smooth and soothe.

• Body lotion: this is your single most important body-treatment product after cleanser. It protects vital moisture and adds a sleek, silky feel to skin, making it comfortable. Smooth lotion on while skin is still damp, to prevent dehydration. Body lotions are usually rich and nongreasy, so that skin feels supple but not weighted down with cream. Some, of course, are richer than others; you may have to experiment until you find those that work best for you.

• Dusting powder or talc: cools and smoothes skin, absorbing moisture so that skin is not irritated. Try one in your favorite scent to help fragrance last.

• Body masks and scrubs: strictly speaking, these are not après-bath products; rather, they can be used anytime. They are, however, particularly efficient when skin is softened from the bath, although they have to be rinsed off with water. Body masks and scrubs cleanse off the layer of dead dry cells at the skin's surface so that new younger and fresher cells can replace it, and they stimulate circulation, too, in much the same way friction mitts and loofahs do, but their action is often gentler because they are cream- or oil-based. There are many on the market, but this is one you can whip up in a blender yourself. The recipe is from Lydia Sarfati of the Klisar Skin Care Center, who recommends it for polishing even the delicate skin of your breasts and abdomen:

Almond and Honey Body Mask

1½ lb. almonds	½ lb. raw oatmeal
4 oz. honey	1 pint buttermilk

Combine all and blend to a thick, smooth paste. Rub over skin and leave on for 20 minutes. Rinse off in a tepid shower and follow with a layer of body lotion.

BATHING TO RELAX

The bath has a history of pleasing the senses while preserving beauty. Some four thousand years ago, Minoan queens spent hours in tiled bathrooms. Cleopatra, like all fine Egyptian ladies, luxuriated in milk and perfumed waters. The Greeks believed that baths drove sadness from the mind and indulged frequently, as did the Romans who made an orgy of it all. Actually, though, through the ages baths had their ups and downs. Elizabeth I of England, for example, bathed only once a month, while Marie Antoinette got into the tub in a flannel nightshirt, believing nakedness was a sin; something that felt so good had to be bad. But now we know better. Beyond cleansing, bathing is conducive to relaxation, tranquillity, and relief from tension.

The bath that does the most good for you should not last more than fifteen minutes, say the experts. Water should be comfortably warm, because it's most calming to muscles and mind, and allows cleansers and other bath products to perform the way they were designed to. A too long, too hot soak will dissolve protective surface oils, your skin's main lines of defense against the drying environment, permitting you to lose moisture through perspiration. Skin wrinkles and puckers. Very hot water can be dangerous too—for anyone who is overweight or has circulatory problems—as is a bath that's too cold and shocks the system. Any extremes of temperature should be approached gradually, and perhaps approved by your physician beforehand.

If problem-solving is your goal, however, before you try anything else, give the following water therapy a chance:

• *Problem:* tension. *Solution:* relax in warm bubbly water, letting your head roll in circles to release tension in your neck and shoulders. Then stretch out, leaning your head on a pillow so you're submerged from the neck down. Close your eyes for several minutes, then begin cleansing.

• *Problem:* achy muscles. *Solution:* sit in a warm bath, gradually adding hotter water. Then attach a rubber hose to your faucet and direct a jet of water over sore areas while they are submerged.

• *Problem:* sunburn and chapping. *Solution:* relax in a warm bath for several minutes, then add bath oil. Let cooler water slowly trickle in. Do not cleanse. When you get out of the tub, blot skin lightly, then add moisturizer to the film of oil already on your body.

• *Problem:* insomnia. *Solution:* begin with warm water and bubbles, adding hot water gradually. Before you go to bed, your bath can be hotter; the effect is more soporific. Laze under a blanket of bubbles, sipping warm milk. Gently blot dry. Then smooth on powder and moisturizer and slip between clean sheets.

Exercising in the tub has very beneficial effects; water creates resistance, so you get more out of every movement. Sit on a rubber mat though to keep from sliding:

• To strengthen arms and legs: sit straight up in the tub with your legs extended and hands under buttocks, turning fingers in. Push up, keeping arms and legs straight, lifting body up and off the bottom of the tub. Relax back down and repeat 4 times.

• To strengthen stomach and abdomen: sit up with legs together and straight. Extend arms overhead and bend from the hips until your nose almost touches the

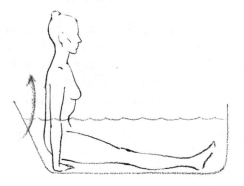

water. Return to an upright position and slowly repeat 4 times.

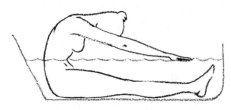

• To strengthen thighs: lean back in the tub with your head on a pillow and your arms at your sides with legs extended. Bend your left knee, keeping your left foot flat, and raise your right leg—knee straight—then lower it, 5 times. Change legs and repeat.

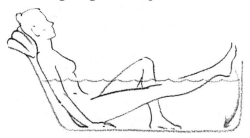

SHOWERING TO REENERGIZE

In winter, when your skin is dry and too much soaking depletes natural moisture, or in summer, when you want to rinse off repeatedly during the day without stripping your skin, hop into the shower. It gives a quick, reenergizing lift and uses only one tenth the amount of water a bath would—three gallons to a bath's thirty gallons.

Keep the water warm, not hot, and if you can, attach a pulsating shower-head that allows you to adjust the water intensity. If you're feeling especially tired, gradually run water cooler, finishing with a cool—but not cold—rinse. Be sure to place a nonskid mat in the tub to prevent accidents.

Unwind even further by taking the kinks out of your shoulders while you're standing under a strong massaging stream of water:

• direct the spray on your right shoulder. Lift it and rotate it clockwise 5 times, then counterclockwise 5 times. Switch spray to your left shoulder and repeat.

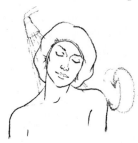

• put your hands on your chest, spreading your fingers, and try to raise your elbows to shoulder level. Rotate them 10 times clockwise, then 10 times counterclockwise.

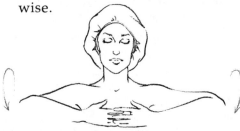

As soon as you leave the shower, stroke body cream or lotion over your damp skin, massaging it firmly to speed up skin's circulation.

THE PROFESSIONAL MASSAGE

Massage has a place in every busy woman's life. It's certainly one of the pleasantest ways to unwind. "It has both beauty and therapeutic benefit," explains Lydia Sarfati. "It increases the circulation, and that's important for the woman after forty," continues Lydia, "because the blood can then more efficiently carry away waste products so that the skin tone and color is improved." Massage does not replace daily exercising; it works with it. By soothing the muscles, it relaxes the nerves, too, allowing you to detense totally.

There are many different kinds of massage; every masseur or masseuse seems to have his or her own method, sometimes employing Shiatsu techniques, which consist of manipulation of pressure points—the same ones used in acupuncture—to relax and relieve aches, as well as Swedish massage—a combination of stroking, rubbing, kneading, and tapping, which may vary from very light to heavy, depending on the area being worked. All strokes, however, are rhythmic and slow, and fingers can be speeded along with a rub of oil or rich cream, so the effect is pleasant. "I don't believe that a massage should hurt," says Lydia, "regardless of differences in delivery. If a massage is painful and unpleasant, you cannot relax. To be effective, pressure should not be too heavy—or too light. It has to feel comfortable. You want to be both stimulated and relaxed at the same time." How can you judge a massage? "If you feel that all tension has left you, and you either fall asleep or feel revived after your session, I'd say your massage was a good one."

SAUNAS AND STEAM BATHS

These high-heat treatments soothe and purify the skin, unknot muscles, and help to drain tension. Most important, though, says Dr. Kantor, "They add moisture to the skin. But you have to be healthy to withstand them. Anyone with cardiovascular or lung problems should avoid them."

Both saunas and steam baths encourage you to perspire—and this perspiration serves to cleanse the skin. In addition, the heat stimulates circulation, improving color. Follow both with a tepid shower, then lock in moisture with a film of body lotion, applied lavishly to still-damp skin.

WHAT TO DO ABOUT BODY HAIR

The skin you love to touch is soft, smooth—and probably free of unwanted hair. If it's not, no problem. Body hair is relatively easy to mini-mize or get rid of—by bleaching, waxing, shaving, tweezing, or electrolysis. The process you use should be determined by the area of your body, as well as by the time, effort, and cost involved. You'll notice too that nature will help, because after menopause pubic and underarm hair get sparser.

For quick reference, here's a matchup of body spots and the most effective ways of removing hair found in each:

Forearms—bleaching is a good choice if hair is fine; depilatories and waxing are also effective if hair is coarse. Do not shave.

Breasts—tweezing or clipping stray hairs with a pair of little scissors are temporary solutions. Electrolysis is permanent.

Bikini line—shaving and waxing are both options, although both can be irritating and waxing can result in ingrown hairs. Electrolysis is effective, but it can be very time-consuming and costly if you have a lot of hair.

Stomach—bleach, wax, or use a depilatory on darker fuzz. Tweezing and electrolysis are fine, but only if you have a few coarse hairs.

Legs—shaving, depilatories, and waxing are all acceptable: electrolysis is very impractical for the legs. If you have varicose veins, avoid waxing, because the stress on the skin and veins from pulling could aggravate this condition.

The basic techniques themselves

vary in cost, effort, comfort, and longevity:

• *Bleaching*—lightens dark hair, making it less obvious. Bleaching works best on fair skin because hair will then blend into the skin tones; bleached blond body hair may look unnatural on skin that's dark or olive. Since this process is sometimes irritating, take a patch test. Bleach should always be applied to skin that's first washed with cold water so pores are closed, then dried. If water is hot, pores will open and skin will become more sensitive. Bleaching lasts until the hair grows out and replaces itself.

• *Chemical depilatories*—leave skin slightly smoother than shaving, for a slightly longer time—about a week—because they dissolve the hair below the surface. They are best for large areas but can be irritating, so a patch test is recommended. Depilatories are available in foam, cream, and lotion form.

• *Shaving*—the fastest, easiest, and most inexpensive way to remove hair. It does, however, quickly grow back and with a stubbly feel. (Contrary to common misconception, it does not grow back thicker—it just feels thicker because edges are blunted.) The best way to shave is against the hair growth—from the ankle to the knee. If skin gets irritated, try shaving down the leg instead.

• *Waxing*—pulls the hairs out from below the skin line, like tweezing, so that skin is left smooth. Regrowth is finer, and waxing lasts for several weeks—usually from three to eight—depending on how fast hair naturally grows. It can be painful and irritating, though, and leaves skin temporarily reddened. You can wax your legs yourself using one of the packaged waxing kits (hot wax is most efficient), but it's best to leave your underarms and bikini line to a professional. Ingrown hairs, if you are prone to them, commonly accompany waxing since the hair growing under the surface can double back on itself. If they are a problem, buff the area lightly each day with an abrasive surface—a loofah, sponge, or friction mitt—then smooth on body lotion.

• *Electrolysis*—is the only permanent method of hair removal and must be performed by a trained expert. You should never under any circumstances do it yourself, anywhere on your body. It can be painful, expensive, and time-consuming—making it best suited for small areas only.

NAIL CARE

Fingernails can make or break a beauty; they are always on display and an important part of your total look. This does not mean that your nails have to be an inch long and brilliantly polished; they simply need to be groomed. Length, of course, is a matter of choice, but nails risk looking clawlike if too long—and that's dating in addition to being unattractive. Keeping your nails neat and polished is a good idea at every age, but now especially, because nail growth slows down so a break takes even longer to grow out and nails themselves become brittler, thus more disposed to split and peel. Polish helps to strengthen your nails and protect them; regular manicures keep your nails in shape. If you are not in a position to have professional manicures, here's how you can care for your nails in the gentlest possible way.

Give yourself a lasting manicure

Begin by assembling all the tools you'll need: a fine emery board or diamond-dust metal file, an orange stick, cuticle clippers, cotton, oily nail polish remover (oil helps to offset the drying effects of acetone, the main ingredient in removers), cuticle remover, liquid soap or detergent, a small bowl, tissues, base coat, nail enamel, top coat, hand cream, and a towel. Now, follow these steps:

• Remove old polish by saturating a cotton pad with remover, pressing it to your nail for several seconds to soften polish, then stroking it off from your cuticle toward the tip of your nail.

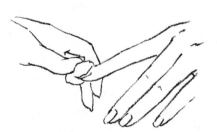

• Shape your nails by filing them lightly from the sides to the centers, in one direction only. Never file in nail corners, leave these straight for support and strength, but round the nail tips.

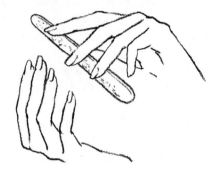

• Soften your cuticles by soaking your fingertips in warm, sudsy water for several minutes.

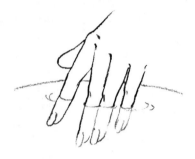

• Blot your fingers, apply cuticle remover, then push cuticles gently back with an orange stick. Do not

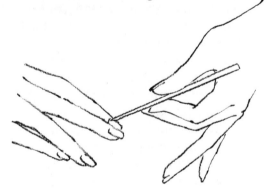

apply too much pressure, because you can damage the living part of the nail, located under the cuticle.

• With the edge of your towel wipe off remover and dead skin, while pushing cuticles back again.

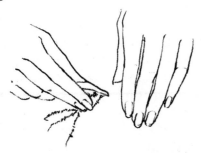

• Lightly trim any ragged edges, using the points of your clippers.

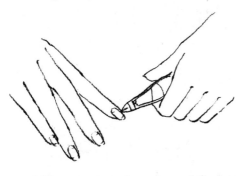

• Massage your hands and fingers with lotion, then wipe any cream residue off your nails with cotton dipped in sudsy water. Dry nails carefully, again pushing cuticles back.

• Stroke on two coats of base—it prevents nails from discoloring from the polish that follows and helps the polish adhere.

• Apply two coats of polish. The color you select depends on your coloring, clothing, your mood. Best is a shade that complements your skin tone. If you have brown spots on the backs of your hands, stay away from bright colors that call attention to your hands. One trick to see how a color looks on you without disturbing your manicure is to take a roll of clear tape with you when you're shopping. In the store, place a small piece on your hand and apply nail color to it. When you get outside, check to see how the color works with your skin. Clear nail enamel is only a good idea if your nails are very white and smooth, and if your coloring is not too pale. Most hands look best now with a bit of color.

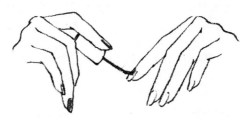

• Dip your orange stick in remover and clean away smudges.

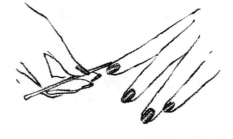

• Finish with a top coat to protect polished surface.

Nail-saving tips

• Don't change your polish more than once a week—remover is very drying.

• Give a few-days-old manicure new life with a thin coat of clear polish or top coat.

• If filling in a chip with a touch-up of polish looks unnatural, try dampening the ball of your finger with remover, rubbing it over the edges of the chip until they are smoothed into the surrounding polish, then covering all with a fresh coat of polish.

• Paler flesh tones can make short nails look longer and short hands more graceful.

• Save your nails by dialing the telephone with a pencil instead of your finger, using a knife to open letters and packages, using the pads of your fingers, rather than your nails, to pick up anything.

• Keep your polish in the refrigerator. It will not thicken as quickly, and application will be smoother.

• Stroke polish on slowly, to avoid bubbles.

• Try to save a nail that's breaking with a nail patch, available in use-at-home kits.

• Quick-dry your manicure by plunging your fingertips into ice-cold water or by brushing them with a specially formulated drying product. Then let polish set for at least a half hour.

• If your nails are soft, use a nail hardener, but sparingly, and on nail tips only. It can cause an allergic reaction; if overused, it can make nails brittle.

• Your cuticles protect the nail bed from infection; they should be clipped only if they are ragged.

• If you pinch a nail, raise your hand to keep blood from rushing to the area, then apply a cold compress.

• Your nails grow slightly faster in hot weather, and when circulation is improved from typing, playing the piano, and massaging your fingers.

• Always wear rubber gloves when washing dishes, doing housework, coloring your hair.

• Cream your nails every night, in dry weather especially, to keep them, and the skin around them, supple.

YOUR HANDS

The skin on your hands ages faster than your face, because it's extremely thin, with less subcutaneous tissue (padding below the skin) than almost any other exposed body part. It's at the mercy of the elements—sun, water, wind, and cold—as well as everything else you handle. It needs protection to stay soft and smooth.

Use a rich hand lotion before you do anything, and after as well. A silicone-based product is particularly helpful if your activity is water-related, like swimming. Then wear gloves when washing dishes, gardening, and the like. Rubber gloves with a cotton lining are a good choice, because the cotton absorbs moisture. But since wetness can lead to a bacteria or fungus buildup, always turn your gloves inside out to dry. Protect hands from the sun with a sunscreen, and whenever they feel especially dry and chapped, smear petroleum jelly over them and sleep with white cotton gloves.

The brown spots you might see on the backs of your hands are changes in pigment due to age and/or sun exposure. Sometimes they respond to a bleaching solution prescribed by your dermatologist. And most can be removed surgically, with an electric needle or deep peeling, in the same manner as they are removed from the face. Although a procedure exists for pulling excess and wrinkled skin taut, flattening out veins, it is very complicated and rarely performed. Called a hand lift, it leaves a marked scar along the top of the wrist.

If your hands swell after you have been sitting for a while, it could be because of a compression in your shoulder, being overweight, sitting stiffly so that shoulder and upper-arm muscles press against the veins, poor posture, or a tight bra strap. After you remedy these causes, gloves that exert pressure on the hands, forcing fluids back to the tissues, are helpful in lessening swelling. Avoid compressing or rupturing veins by carrying heavy packages with a handle rather than a thin string, so that pressure is evenly distributed over the hands.

YOUR FEET

The skin on the tops of your feet is very thin too, and dry, like the backs of your hands, while the soles are thicker. Moisturize feet every day with rich lotion, preferably after bathing, while they're still damp.

Your feet are under a lot of stress—and if you're overweight, this pressure is even more intense—on only three weight-bearing points: the heel and the two metatarsal bones found under the big and the little toes. If your shoes do not fit well, if your heels are too high, if your posture is not up to par, you can develop corns and calluses. Corns should always be professionally removed, as should those calluses that are not smoothed by daily pumicing in the bath or shower. To keep your feet comfortable, experts suggest wearing a heel of between one and a half and one and three-quarters inches during the day and caution against changing heel heights too frequently, or too quickly, because it strains your calf muscles.

When feet are hot and tired, massage them with creams containing menthol—they cool and soothe. Massage boosts circulation and revitalizes the important nerve-endings located in the soles of your feet. Always smooth a generous amount of cream over the area you are massaging, so that your fingers can slide over the skin. Complete the whole massage on one leg before switching to the other:

Step 1—warm up the calf area by stroking it for several minutes. Do this by applying pressure with your thumbs and fingers, working up toward the heart—from your ankles to your knees.

Step 3—increase flexibility by rotating each toe slowly.

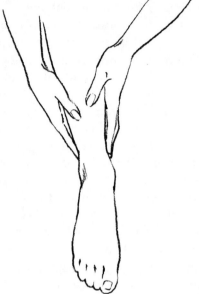

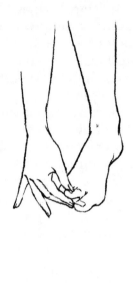

Step 2—step up sluggish circulation by massaging between toes in a circular motion, using your thumb.

Step 4—stroke and massage the foot area only, using the same motions as in step 1.

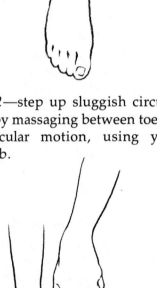

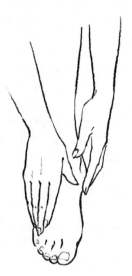

Step 5—apply pressure with your thumbs, using circular movements, and massage around your ankle bone.

As often as necessary, try lubricating your feet with a coat of petroleum jelly massaged all over, covered by a pair of white cotton socks and left on overnight.

Keeping your feet fit

• When feet get cramped and weary and you don't have a minute for a massage, try this two-step exercise for a refreshing pause: First flex feet and toes, then round feet and curl toes under as far as they will go. Repeat 4 times.

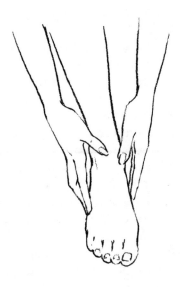

Step 6—again using your thumbs, manipulate the sole of your foot. Work from the heel to the instep and then the ball of the foot, maintaining firm pressure in a slow, steady movement.

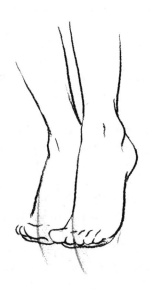

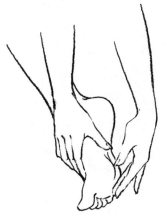

• If you're on your feet often, walk barefoot sometimes, but only on soft or grassy surfaces. Also, slip into clogs, because they help reinforce the arches of the feet without any effort so that ligaments are not stressed and tired.

• Take off your shoes from time to time during the day to give feet a breather.

• Feet swell when you sit for a long time—on airplanes especially. Flex your feet and stretch them if you can't walk around for a little while.

• Avoid pointed-toe shoes. They can crowd the toes and cause corns.

• Another tired-feet reviver: run cold water over your feet for 2 minutes, then hot water, then cold again, and repeat 3 times.

• Always wear the correct footgear when you are jogging or running—special shoes made for these sports cushion the feet the way ordinary sneakers cannot.

• While bunions are not hereditary, the tendency to develop them is inherited. If you have bunions but no pain, simply buy shoes a little wider. If your bunions hurt, consult your physician. Today there are many surgical techniques to deal with bunions, some relatively simple.

• Make sure your panty hose or stockings are long enough, to keep your feet healthy and problem-free. There should be about half an inch to spare in your toes. Always pull out the toes before putting on your shoes.

The professional pedicure

A pedicure can help keep your feet pretty, pampered, and comfortable. A professional one is best—with a top-notch expert—since it's sometimes difficult to bend over and get at the right angle to groom your feet yourself. However, it can be done; give yourself a pedicure once every month and try to cream your feet daily. Your toenails do not have to match your fingernails, but keep the colors in the same family.

Begin your pedicure by assembling everything you need, exactly as you did for a manicure, substituting a pan for the small bowl and adding a pair of toenail clippers. The best time to give yourself a pedicure is after a bath or shower, so that your skin is softened.

• Remove old polish.

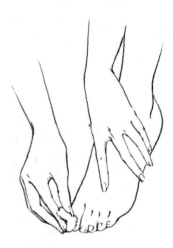

• Clip nails straight across, slightly shorter than the ends of your toes. If you cut them too short, or too far back at the corners, you risk ingrown nails.

• Take your bath or shower—or soak feet in warm, sudsy water—smoothing calluses and rough spots with a pumice stone. Never cut them with any kind of implement; see a podiatrist if they bother you.

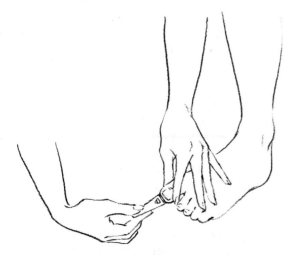

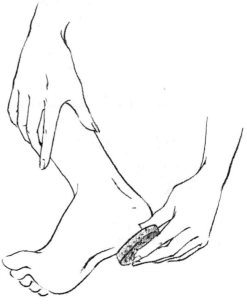

• File nails lightly, slightly rounding sharp corners.

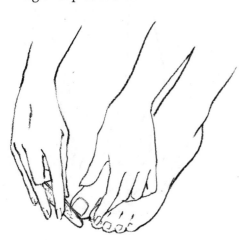

• Apply cuticle remover, then push cuticles gently back with an orange stick.

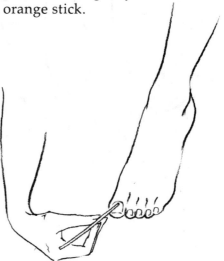

• With a towel, wipe nails clean, pushing cuticles back again.

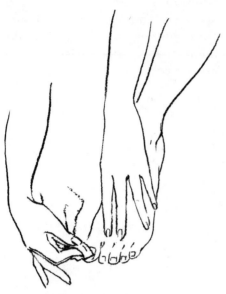

• Cream feet and toes with body lotion.

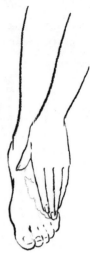

• Trim any ragged cuticles with your cuticle clippers.

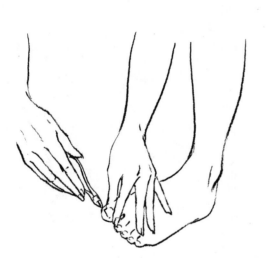

• Wipe cream residue from nails, using a dampened cotton ball, then dry nails thoroughly.

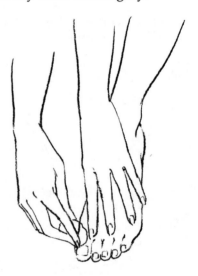

• Separate toes by weaving a folded tissue through them.

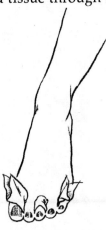

• Apply two coats of base coat, then two coats of color. Clean smudges with an orange stick dipped in remover. Finish with a thin layer of top coat.

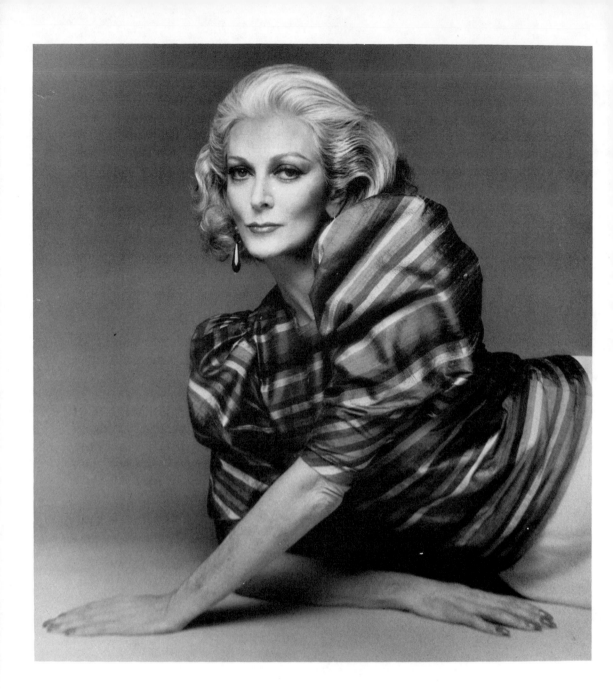

Carmen

Model

It took me a long time to give myself permission to take myself from last place on the list—in other words, to allow myself pleasure. But that's one sure strength I see in myself that's come with maturity. Also, I have the ability to spend my energies with more efficiency. The only way I'd want to be twenty again is if I could take with me the knowledge I now have. I mean, if I could be the person I am today, with all the experience I have—and not have to repeat the thirty years from twenty to fifty.

I feel, in terms of goals, that until one achieves the centeredness of feeling good and knowing how one works day in and day out, one has nothing to offer. I want to find out how best to give and receive love, and this is only done by interacting with people and society.

I had a very unusual life, though, and didn't go through the same kind of process as a lot of women. I began working young and had responsibility early. I had very strong goals then, that I had to give up. I had to learn to be flexible and adjust to disappointment. I wanted to be a ballet dancer, had a scholarship for the Ballet Russe, but had to stop because I contracted rheumatic fever. I began swimming for therapy and became quite proficient because I had enormous drive and discipline from ballet, as well as natural grace in the water. I began swimming competitively but broke my leg skiing two weeks before the Olympics. So, at age fourteen, I began modeling—and quite by accident. I was discovered on a bus. But the initial photographs didn't turn out well, and my mother has a classic letter saying that I was a charming and well-mannered child, but unfortunately, unphotogenic. And that sent me into another disappointment—I didn't know the word "depression" at the time. But my godparents disagreed and sent me to someone they know at **Vogue**. I had seven full pages published within months of the first rejection. Incredible. So, you never know what is going to happen. You can't let things get you down. Easy to say, I know, but difficult to implement emotionally. The only way to survive is to not want anything—to keep going, to learn not to be angry. If something good happens, well then, that's marvelous. If you absorb anger and retain resentments, I think this leads to disease.

Well, after the initial **Vogue** encounter, my career was set. I then retired in 1966—stayed home with my daughter, decorated, painted, and did all the things I wanted. My life luckily afforded me the opportunity to do them. My husband said that I didn't have to work if I didn't want to. But truly, I never worked *as hard as when I stayed home! I decided to return to modeling in 1980—and I feel good about myself, and the way I look.*

My fitness routine is so built in that my first instinct is to deny doing anything. But I do—I exercise every day. In bed, I stretch and do sit-ups in the morning. I find that this helps right my eyesight so that my glasses work when I put them on. If I just reach over upon awakening and put them on, I think my prescription is wrong, and it's because my circulation isn't moving. Most important—I have to move, move, move. I walk everywhere, and I swim all the time. Swimming is the most well-rounded exercise for my body. And it makes me feel wonderful, totally relaxed. It doesn't suit my nature to work out with machines.

I eat when I'm hungry; and if I'm not hungry, I don't eat. If anything, I have to eat to keep my weight up and to have energy. If I don't, I sleep—sleep then becomes my energy source. Basically, I eat red meat once or twice a week—I am not part of this non-meat-eating generation. My diet is balanced—a salad and green vegetables daily. A potato almost every day. And if I don't have my oatmeal in the morning, I can't make it until lunchtime.

I found that after forty I was beginning to know so much about myself that a lot of tensions I had been living with left, so that my skin has never looked better. When I was in my late thirties, I started taking vitamins E, C, and the B's. I find myself very balanced mentally and physically. I don't know how much the vitamins have to do with it, or whether it's that I'm not that organizationally rigid. I'm flexible with my life. I feel that vitamin E has helped my skin, though. I began by taking a couple of hundred IUs daily, worked up to 1,000 and now, 2,000. I generally take 1,000 mg. of C and in the colder weather, more. I used to have respiratory problems, interesting because I never smoked. But now, at worst, I'll get a cold and have to stay in bed a few days.

I care for my skin by washing it with soap, followed by an astringent, then moisturizer from Dr. Norman Orentreich, which I alternate with mineral oil, which really works for me. There are still times of the month when my skin is patchy, so I put on the oil, let it absorb, and blot it—what's left gives my skin an even base. I protect my face with makeup—essential in New York with all the dirt and soot—which I thoroughly remove every night.

When my hair turned gray, I decided to keep it that way. My facial shadows looked different—I looked better with lighter hair. I started to enhance the gray by frosting it several times a year. It looks livelier. People don't know if I am gray, silver, blonde, or whatever. And I like that, too. I like being a little mysterious. My hair texture is easier to style now—I had always such straight hair. But I find that as I have gotten older, I have half the hair I used to on my head, and twice as much on my chin!

I believe in plastic surgery—it's a wonderful advantage available to women. I haven't needed it, but if I did, I would do anything to make myself feel good. And nobody has to give me permission anymore—that's one of the nice things about experience. And I say experience, not aging, because some people age and never learn from experience.

Sure, there's a genetic change involved with aging—the system goes through a gradual process of breaking down. But there is a mental attitude about it that is either "up" or "down." And I am an "up" person—I try to have a sense of humor about it all. As my perspective grows, there is more to enjoy. Life is funnier, better, bigger, richer. It's more everything, and that's why I wouldn't go back in time.

Part V

For Body and Soul

Chapter 15

Using Fragrance to Your Psychological Advantage

You want to look smashing now and feel that way too. And interestingly enough, fragrance can help by giving you a psychological advantage: emotional satisfaction. For fragrance is known to change moods, lift spirits—even overcome depression! "Odors provoke strong emotional responses because the areas of the brain devoted to smell and emotion overlap," explains Dr. Susan Schiffman, associate professor of medical psychology, Duke University Medical Center. She explains that when the cortex was forming, it was first totally devoted to smell, then this early part later developed into the seat of the emotions as well.

"Fragrance can help you feel better and thus look better in whatever way you want at the time; when you smell something you like, you feel happier," claims Bernard Chant, senior vice-president and chief perfumer of International Flavors & Fragrances. "We believe that the sense of smell is very much attached to memories, and fragrances can revive past pleasures and joys." He continues that in his opinion no fragrances are youthful or aging, they have to do with your own perception of yourself. "You see in a fra-grance certain things that you like in life; you should use those scents that correspond to your life-style and activities—to what you are, not how old you are," he emphasizes.

What can be aging, however, is fragrance rigidity, growing so set in your ways that you stay with the same scent through the years. You're depriving yourself of a full range of emotions, of new experiences that you could be receiving when you experiment with scents—plus, you're probably not even benefiting from the full emotional impact of the scent you've been wearing because of "nose fatigue"; when you get used to a scent, you can no longer even smell it. Mr. Chant suggests exploring new scents every three months to match your mood at the time, or refresh it. Then you can always return to your special or "signature" scent from time to time or for certain occasions.

Especially now, it's very important to explore the world of scent, because experimentation may actually help you to offset any decline in your sense of smell—the first sense to show a deterioration with age. Some experts place the figure at an early thirty-five, others later, but sometime in your middle years your ability to detect smells and to distinguish between them begins to decline very gradually.

However, the thinking is that you may help to retard this decline by actively using your sense of smell throughout your life. Dr. Schiffman points out that older perfumers have a significantly better ability to distinguish and discriminate odors than other older subjects as an indication that the concept "use it or lose it" may apply to smell as it does to so many of the other physical functions.

AROMATHERAPY AS EMOTIONAL THERAPY

Just why certain scents have certain effects in the psyche is attributed by the experts to association. And when these associations are pleasant, they say, you have a feeling of well-being. Vanilla can be considered comforting because of its association with the aroma of fresh-baked cookies, citrus notes are revitalizing because they recall orange juice in the morning. If you think back through literature, scent and emotion are strongly linked—Marcel Proust's total recall of an earlier,

happier, and totally forgotten time was released the moment he smelled a freshly baked little cake, a madeleine. Through the ages man has called upon scent to help him—first for prayer, then for personal adornment and psychological enhancement.

The concept of aromatherapy—therapy through the sense of smell—is receiving attention these days as experts look toward scent to help make life healthier, happier, to help us deal with the stresses we encounter. But aromatherapy as emotional therapy may involve a reaction that's more than psychological; it could be chemical. Perfume's power to seduce, for example. We know that scent plays an important part in the courtship and mating of animals, and scientists are currently investigating whether pheromones, the chemical substances secreted by animals and insects to trigger the opposite sex, exist in humans and whether they can be applied in perfume form. Although we know that fragrance plays a role in our relationships, it's usually on a more unconscious level and used to trigger emotions, not instincts. As of now, results are inconclusive, but progress appears to be promising.

That certain scents have specific emotional effects cannot be denied; the proof is in the spraying! Here are a few of the notes celebrated in herbal lore for their mood-modification abilities—but, of course, the way they are blended in your personal perfume can influence the final effect. Some, you'll notice, can soothe *and* stimulate—so experiment with them.

Specific Scents and Their Effects

Notes that calm you down:

bergamot	lily of the valley
camomile	narcissus
camphor	rose
geranium	sandalwood
honeysuckle	vanilla
hyacinth	ylang-ylang
lavender	

Notes that pick you up:

basil	lavender
citrus	patchouli
clove	peppermint
cypress	rose
geranium	sandalwood
jasmine	ylang-ylang

Notes that bolster your confidence:

geranium	vetiver
lavender	ylang-ylang
sandalwood	

Notes that give you energy:

jasmine	rosemary
juniper	tuberose
patchouli	

Perfumes and Their Powers
(What you can expect from the perfume you wear)

Scents that soothe:

Adolfo	Calandre
Amazone	Chloë
Arpège	L'Air du Temps
Bill Blass	Maja
	Murasaki

Scents that stimulate:

Bal à Versailles	Miss Dior
Calvin Klein	Opium
Cie	Quartz
Joy	White Linen

Ego-boosting scents:

Alexandra	Complice de Coty
Cardin de Pierre Cardin	J'ai Osé
Chanel No. 5	Shalimar
Chantilly	Vôtre

HOW FRAGRANCE HAS HELPED MAN THROUGH THE AGES

While the term might be modern, the concept of aromatherapy is both ancient and divine. The first man-made perfumes were a by-product of the discovery of fire. Early man noticed that burning woods and gums gave off odors—in fact, the word "perfume" is derived from the Latin "per," or "through," and "fumus," meaning "smoke." Fire was mystical to him and smoke sacred, so he used scented smoke as a messenger to carry his prayers to heaven. Since he enjoyed the smell, he believed the gods did as well.

Later man realized that perfume did not have to be made with fire but could be composed in waters and oils that could then be rubbed on the body. He began to take advantage of the scented pleasures that up until now had been reserved for the gods.

Priests in ancient Egypt used aromatics during religious ceremonies and mummification rites to ward off evil spirits; physicians used them to help heal the sick, and Egyptian women perfumed their bodies to seduce their lovers. Cleopatra was one of the most famous scent-users; she supposedly fragranced herself and her barge with roses to win the love and political influence of Mark Antony.

During their long captivity in Egypt the Hebrews learned the arts of perfumery, which they used primarily for holy purposes, although Judith, a Jewish heroine who saved her native city by seducing the besieging Assyrian commander, used perfume to aid her. The Greeks learned much about the properties and uses of aromatics from the Egyptians and also believed in their divine origins, attributing the invention of perfumes to the gods. It was recognized by the Greeks that aromatic plants, flowers, especially, had either a stimulative or sedative effect, and it was their custom, if they were wealthy, to anoint different parts of their bodies with different scents—men were as luxuriously perfumed as women.

The Romans were yet more lavish in their use of scent—perfuming their hair, bodies, clothes, beds, walls, even military flags. They also massaged with perfumed oils to heal and soothe body and spirit. With the decline of the Roman empire, perfume passed to the East—the Byzantines and the Arabs. It was at the end of the tenth century that an Arabian physician invented modern perfume by distillation—extracting the essential oil from a flower. His discovery—rosewater—was brought to Europe along with other exotic essences and perfumes during the Crusades, and enterprising businessmen found more profit in manufacturing their own scents than in importing them.

In about 1370, Hungary Water distilled from rosemary became the vogue. Purportedly created by Queen Elizabeth of Hungary, who received the secret of its preparation from an old hermit, the scent made her so desirable that men were taken with her charms when she was seventy; at age seventy-two, still irresistible, she was asked by the king of Poland to marry him.

During the Middle Ages scent was universally popular at court—in Italy and England, then in France. But perfumes of those times would hardly be recognized as such today—they were overwhelmingly pungent. It was perhaps Madame de Pompadour who helped change the trend from primarily heavy Eastern scents to more delicate floral ones like hyacinth, her favorite. Marie Antoinette adopted this attitude and popularized the pleasures of the perfumed bath. Napoleon's wife Josephine also preferred simple, natural scents like violet and jasmine.

Early in the eighteenth century the classic eau de cologne, based on citrus notes, was a best seller and continues to this day as a fragrance staple, particularly in Europe. During the nineteenth century toilet waters, rather than perfumes, were worn, as anything too strong was considered cheap. Of course, during all this time essential oils continued to be a mainstay in medicines and potions, in cosmetics and creams—the roots of today's aromatherapy.

FACTORS THAT AFFECT YOUR FRAGRANCE REACTION

The mood-altering abilities of fragrance helped us cope with life in the past and continue to do likewise at present, in ways we may not totally understand. But in order to get what you want from the fragrance you wear, you must first consider the factors that affect your reaction.

• Your age: the gradual decline in the sense of smell with age can sometimes result in heavy fragrance application. And when the fragrance is a potent one, the combination is often overwhelming. Fragrance should suggest, never shout, and you do not have to be able to smell it on yourself to know that it's there. If you like an intense scent, apply less of it or use a lighter variation, toilet water instead of perfume.

• Your skin type: fragrance lasts a shorter time on dry skin—because it absorbs the oils almost immediately—than it does on oily skin. If your skin is drier, and it probably will be, since oil production declines with age, experiment with complex scents that have more body and staying power.

• Your emotional state: high-strung, emotional, and sensitive types—whether by nature or as a result of changes at midlife—have a harder time "holding" scent; body heat and glandular secretions generated by high emotions move fragrance off the skin, and fast. To keep it in place, you should reapply scent more often, so select a lighter, fresher variety that won't become overpowering through frequent application and will help cool down your temperament at the same time.

• Your environment: fragrance flowers best and lasts longest in a hot, humid climate, least and shortest in dry cold. So switch scents with the seasons, keeping the lightest, verviest fragrances for those times when the temperature is highest.

• Your diet: change your diet, and your skin's reaction to your scent will change as well. Oily, spicy, and rich foods, as well as some fish, cause odors to come through the pores, resulting in an imbalance with the fragrance you're wearing, so that it may smell "off."

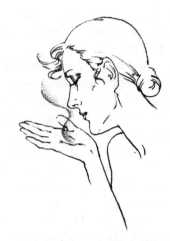

and you'll have difficulty differentiating between them since the nose gets confused; check your reaction to them throughout the day.

SHOPPING FOR SCENT

You can't determine how a fragrance will smell on you by sniffing it in the bottle—or on the wrist of a salesperson. And even when you try it on, it takes time for the fragrance to blend with your skin oils—anywhere from ten minutes to an hour—so that the initial note, or top note, gives way to the heart, the full character of the scent.

It's best to shop for scent in the late afternoon, because your sense of smell becomes keener as the day goes on. If you're feeling particularly tense, take a sample home with you to try when you are calmer, since nerves affect blood vessels, thus your sense of smell. Test scent by spraying one cologne or toilet water over your right palm and another over your left—the heat and perspiration will help to release the scent, and you'll be able to experience it whenever you lift your hands. Try no more than two or three scents (spray the third on the back of one hand) at a time; more,

HOW TO WEAR FRAGRANCE

"Cologne is meant to refresh, not last; apply it like you would powder after the bath. Toilet water then sets the base, like makeup foundation, while perfume, like lipstick and eye makeup, adds overall impact," explains Annette Green, executive director of the Fragrance Foundation, a nonprofit educational organization concerned with the role of fragrance in our lives. For each form of fragrance should be worn in a special way to extend its pleasures. Those in the know suggest layering scent for longest last—beginning with scented soap and bath oil, then matching body lotion and talc, and finally cologne, toilet water, and perfume.

• *Cologne*—is the lightest form of fragrance and often a diluted version of perfume but less highly concentrated with oils than toilet water. Cologne should be splashed all over the body after the bath or shower to cool your skin and refresh it, as an invigorating pickup on a hot day, too. It also helps keep hands and feet fragrantly cool and dry because its alcohol content aids in evaporating perspiration.

• *Toilet water*—is next in strength and provides an ideal perfume base. It can be worn over or instead of cologne; it can also be used instead of perfume if the scent is too intense in a very concentrated form. You can also "wear" toilet water by spraying it over hair, by adding a few drops to the rinse water after washing lingerie, saturating a piece of cotton and keeping it in the linen closet, and spraying your ironing board before pressing your blouses.

• *Perfume*—is the most concentrated form of fragrance, thus the strongest and longest lasting. A blend of essential oils, natural and/or chemical aromas, plus fixatives and specially aged alcohol that acts as a carrier and determines the final strength, a fine perfume may contain as many as three hundred or more different elements. Apply perfume wherever you feel your pulse beat, so the body heat will help bring out the fragrance, and from the inside of the ankles up, since perfume rises—behind the knees, between the thighs, the bosom, throat, base of the neck, the insides of the wrists, elbows, and behind the ears. If you place it only behind

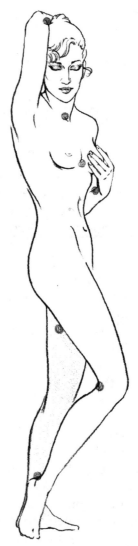

your ears, it will simply rise over your head.

Perfume should be refreshed every few hours, although it will usually linger about six hours. Apply it about an hour before going out so that its true character can develop. Do not save an opened bottle of perfume for special occasions only, because the character of the scent changes with time and exposure to light and air. Keep it in a cool dark place, such as a closet or drawer.

Chapter 16

The Spa Experience

For her fortieth birthday, Cynthia, a high-powered fashion executive, received a week at the Golden Door, one of America's foremost spas, as a gift from her husband. "I realized that I'm out of shape," she explained. "I'm lazy and don't move much. I felt a spa would be a good catalyst; it would show me what to do, then maybe some of what I learned would stick. And since I have a sleeping problem, I thought the exercise would help me sleep." Like a lot of women, Cynthia also believed a spa stay was something she should do for herself. "In the past I was involved almost exclusively with my job and my goals—I worked all the time. But now I'm becoming more aware of myself, what I need to look and feel great. My husband surprised me with this present, but it was one I had wanted for a long time. And I think it was something he wanted me to do as well." She went on, "I feel good about being forty. I see it as a turning point. I consider myself part of a whole era of women who are now more important in society than they were twenty years ago. Part of my positive feeling about my age has to do with the media, though—all of those articles about how beautiful forty is, about those women who are over forty and fab-

ulous, like Jane Fonda. Her body is simply amazing. I look at her and compare myself—if she can do it, so can I."

If you want to make some changes in your life, your looks, but you can't seem to get started, or you don't know where to start, the spa experience can be a marvelous motivation, a first step toward continued improvements. It can give you a new way of seeing yourself and those around you, thus enriching the quality of your life. For many it's a chance to get in touch again with inner feelings and to redirect goals. Explains Deborah Szekely, owner/founder of the Golden Door, "Many of us set our goals at twenty. Come forty, these goals no longer fit. We need to redefine them according to our current needs. Our guest wants to put more beauty—joy, health, appreciation—into her life. She comes here to find the dream, to add the extra dimension. She finds the time to put her head together, sort out problems, and plan how to do things differently. The success of the Door depends on her going home and doing things well. Everyone here contributes to the experience— that's what gives this place its magic." A spa like the Golden Door can help you after forty, like Cynthia, establish the habits that will keep you looking your best at every age.

"For today's woman, her hope chest is her own good health," says Deborah. "If she has any sense, her life should be easier after forty. I believe that you're not only better at forty . . . fifty . . . sixty . . . you are the best! Some things do improve with age—like ultimate values. You concern yourself less with the superficial that takes so much time and energy. And the Door can help you to see what more life has to offer."

So, the reasons why women go to a spa vary. But somewhere among them is the belief that they not only need this time, they deserve it, too. "I read about spas in the magazines," said Cynthia, "but I was always very hostile toward them—because I wasn't informed. I thought they were just for rich women who had nothing else to do. Then a friend who works with me came here, and returned raving about it. She's plain, slim, and did not represent what I thought a spa represented. I revised my thinking, and wanted to go as well. Now I think a spa is something I should do for myself on a regular basis. Maybe this spa every few years, or maybe another."

What makes spa-goers continue the experience in their everyday lives? Let's look beyond the Golden Door's locked gates for an answer. Of course, all spas are not alike—where you go depends on what you want to gain from your stay, and what you want to spend for the experience as well. At the Door the emphasis is on holistic beauty—the mind/body connection. Fitness is key, and food, albeit low-calorie for most, is very important. It is always fresh and nutritious and lovingly presented. "The quality of energy is gotten from the quality of the food," observes Deborah. "Food is the fuel—it's a necessity, but for psychological as well as for physical energy. It can soothe, it can comfort, and it should give sensory pleasure."

ARRIVAL

The grounds are lush, green, and landscaped. The buildings low and graceful, and tastefully decorated in the oriental style. The Golden Door consists of 157 acres of flowering courtyards and outdoor walkways, trees, shrubs, and sand gardens, rippling streams and waterfalls, even a farm that furnishes the fresh-grown organic fruits and vegetables. The staff, cheerfully accommodating and always available, outnumbers the thirty-four guests three to one; your wish is their command.

As soon as you arrive, you are weighed, then measured at thirteen strategic body spots—among them hips, upper thighs, arms, all the places where increased exercise and decreased food intake will really show a change. An interview about your exercise and food preferences follows. While weight loss is not the sole goal, the guests who want to lose pounds are put on a low-calorie diet of, most often, 500 or 700 calories, kicked off by a full day of liquids aptly called Virtue-making Day because guests feel so virtuous about it.

You then return to your room to change for dinner. At the Door all clothing is provided—you need only bring a pair of running shoes, underwear, tights and leotards (they can also be purchased at the boutique), plus a simple outfit for your last evening. In your closet you find a thick white terry robe, slippers, a Japanese-style kimono called a *yukata*, which most of the women wear in the evening, shorts, T-shirts, a jogging outfit, and a raincoat. Everything is laundered daily.

At six thirty you meet for cocktails with the rest of the guests in a small lounge off the dining room. These cocktails—tonight, a delectable mix of juices served hot and garnished with a raspberry—taste far more fattening than their scant 40 calories. A huge bowl of raw vegetables with herb dip is on a low table. You are allowed one of each vegetable. Everyone wears name tags, and chatter is animated. At seven o'clock you are called into the dining room, where you are served a salad composed of greens from the garden, bathed in a zesty dressing that you later learn is a mix of buttermilk, vinegar, dill, and garlic. Fifteen minutes later the entrée arrives—skewered chunks of white meat chicken under a creamy sauce topped with sesame seeds on a bed of crunchy stir-fried vegetables. You are encouraged to eat slowly, and dinner is always served at least forty minutes after cocktails because it takes that long for the stomach to feel full, thus cutting any ravenous hunger when you do eat, so you'll be less likely to feast on bread and butter.

"I come here to get back into good habits," states the woman sitting next to you, who returns yearly. "I do follow the diet suggestions and find they really help. Plus I exercise with the tapes I receive when I leave. I come back when I need more reinforcement."

The age of your group is mixed, but the concentration is late thirties–early forties, then mid-fifties. "At those ages when your body needs a tune-up," explains the woman on your other side. Following coffee, tea, or lemonade—drinks are never served with meals but rather following them, because it's believed they wash everything down so you eat too quickly, while interfering with digestive enzymes—every woman introduces herself and tells where she is from. The directress explains the next day's activities, then it's off to the bathhouse for a sleep-inducing session in the Jacuzzi followed by a back massage.

The emphasis at the Golden Door is on fitness forever. "We try to help you see that movement, like food, is not an option; it's a necessity. You have to put more motion into your life to give yourself more time, added years," explains Deborah Szekely. "The aim here is to restore the balance between rest and motion." Classes are graded—easy, moderate, advanced—and run the gamut of simple stretches (with special classes geared for those with low-back problems), strengthening and water exercises, aerobics, weights, yoga, dance, and relaxation techniques. Most of your day is spent on the move.

DAY 1

The telephone rings at 6:00 A.M. With heavy lids you slip into your jogging suit and stumble out the door into the blackness. You meet in the Blue Lounge for tea or coffee, then gather around the pool for ten minutes of easy stretching before your morning walk. You decide on the easier two-mile walk, saving the vigorous three-mile mountain hike for later in the week. By now the sky is light. The pace is brisk through fragrant trails. You notice shafts of sunshine breaking over distant hills. One-half hour later you have breakfast in the dining room with the other newcomers to discuss your schedule in depth. From tomorrow on, though, you'll be served breakfast in your room. You've decided to be virtuous today—you'll be ingesting six liquid mini-meals for a total of 500 calories, plus a 95-calorie mix of bran, seeds, and raisins in the morning for fiber. On your prettily presented tray you find a paper fan listing your activities: continuous exercise plus a daily massage, herbal wrap, and beauty session. You'll receive a manicure and pedicure later in the week. After a glass of grapefruit juice diluted with a little spring water, plus your bran and a cup of herbal tea, you return to your room to put on your tights and leotard. Your first activity is a warm-up stretching class in one of the glass-enclosed rooms suspended over the gardens. The music is slow, the pace relaxed. It feels glorious simply to move.

One-half hour later you step into the pool for water exercises. The air is crisp, but the water is warm and silky. Your instructor starts slowly, then speeds up the rhythm. Water is the ideal exercise-medium—it increases resistance so that your muscles get a double workout, but it puts no strain on your joints. Pushing that volleyball underwater looks deceptively easy, but you can feel those muscles straining. Forty minutes pass in a blur. You take a quick Jacuzzi, an even quicker shower, and meet in the big gym for aerobic dance, called Da Vinci in honor of the artist, because he was the first to design a group of exercises to work the heart. Against the background of rock and roll music, your enthusiastic instructress, who has boundless energy and one of the best bodies you've ever seen, explains about cardiac fitness and the importance of keeping your pulse rate in the right target zone for your age. You take your pulse again, comparing it to the chart on the wall. You're forty and your pulse is 155. On target again, but many women are too high and have to slow down. By the end of the week, you're assured, you'll simply feel the level that's right for you.

Then ten fifty rolls around, the moment everyone is waiting for—juice break. For those on liquids it's a luscious blend of almonds, banana, and low-fat milk, plus a handful of sunflower seeds; for everyone else, a rich potassium broth that tastes like spicy tomato soup served with raw vegetable hors d'oeuvres. No one complains of hunger.

Your hair consultation with stylist/colorist Kurt is also this first day. He explains that the most prevalent problem he confronts is over-colored, damaged hair. For this he may recommend his nutritious egg-yolk treatment, or his avocado conditioner, or any number of concoctions he whips up in his blender to restore hair beauty. "I also find that many women over forty have too fixed a look—hair that's too done, color that's not realistic. I work with each woman to create a look that fits her life-style, one that's chic and casual during the day and goes dressier at night." You decide to make an appointment for a hair shaping later in the week, and go into the bathhouse for your first blissful herbal bath.

You are wrapped mummy-style (although you can leave your arms out if you wish) in hot sheets scented with rosemary, eucalyptus, and lemon grass; a cold towel is placed over your eyes and forehead. The fragrance soothes the spirit, while the warmth eases tired, sore muscles and helps you perspire away toxins. Low music filters through the room; you're left alone with your thoughts. It's a refreshing pause before spot exercises—those that tighten the abdomen, thighs, backside, trouble spots for most women.

One half-hour of spot exercises passes swiftly. Feeling lither and suppler, you meet with Steve, the only male instructor, in another gym for a session with free weights and machines. "Most women are pear-shaped," he explains. "They have to build and strengthen their upper body, then tighten and tone the lower body to bring it into proportion." You concentrate on upper arms and the muscles supporting your breasts, then your legs, on the machines, which turn out to be far less imposing than you imagined, and a lot more fun.

At 1:00 P.M. lunch is served in brilliant sunshine alongside the pool. Talk turns to expectations about a spa. "I was terribly apprehensive," says a candid woman in her mid-fifties who is forty pounds overweight. "I worried about being accepted. I've put on weight, I haven't been exercising, and I was afraid of being the worst in every class." Another adds, "Women are very critical of their peers, because they're not used to being in groups. Men, though, can just walk into a group and feel right at home. They don't have to undergo scrutiny, they don't even think about not fitting in. Part of the reason I like being here is that it allows me to learn how to be with women." "Being here makes me feel female again," sighs a third. "I'd been so busy redoing my house and before that raising children that I lost sight of who I was." Attention then turns to food. Lunch is a bowl of chilled gazpacho and a handful of sunflower seeds. Someone who chose a high-protein diet is eating a tuna salad. You eat with a demi-tasse spoon, and a little bit goes a very long way.

You relax for a while after lunch before returning to your room for a massage. Accompanied by a tape of soothing music that contains birds twittering, your masseuse kneads the tension out of your body. If any is left, your next activity, called "stretch and relax," eases it fully. Through a series of simple stretches, first at the barre, then down on the floor, you learn how to loosen the muscles you've previously contracted. Then you lie on a mat in the gym, which at this hour is sun-drenched, and let the wonderfully melodious voice of Directress Ann-harriet flow over you, explaining how to unknot every muscle. She covers you with a terry sheet. You drowse until your afternoon juice break—a cucumber/pineapple drink.

At 4:00 P.M. you have yoga. More luxurious stretches that ease your muscles. You learn how to control your breath, your posture, your mind. You feel the life force whirling around you. Enough movement. Now you want to lie still. You have a facial. But first your hands and feet are creamed before being enveloped in heated mitts to help the cream penetrate and soften your skin. Your hair is oiled, then braided and tied with bright yarn ribbons. Finally your skin is analyzed, then creamed with the appropriate preparation, which is formulated at the Golden Door. Your aesthetician explains your week of beauty activities: daily pampering for your hands and feet, different masks and scrubs, a deep pore cleansing, eyebrow tweezing, waxing, lash tinting. Every conceivable beauty service is available, including makeup. You're curious about the celebrities who visit the Door—Robert Wagner and Ali MacGraw, among others. What are they really like? "Nice and friendly," says she. And yes, they do mingle with the other guests.

You drift back to your room—

"high" from all the attention, exercise, and the slight edge of hunger. The cleansing action of the liquids you've been drinking makes you feel instantly thinner, more compact. It's 6:00 P.M. "One part of the Door's uniqueness is that we work our guests an eleven-hour day," explains Deborah. "And if it was not an inherent right of the body, we could not do it. In earlier times man did just that, and we still have the capacity for it. There's an enormous wholeness that comes from using the body completely. You've done what nature intended you to do." You shower before dinner. Cocktails—you wonder what they will be tonight—are in a scant half hour.

The cocktail atmosphere is festive, but some faces are missing—several guests like to dine in their rooms. As one new friend had explained earlier in the day, "I work very hard and when I come here, I'm exhausted. Almost too exhausted to speak. My greatest fear is that I'll meet someone I want to talk to and tire myself further. So for the first few days I purposely avoid encounters and have dinner in my room. My last evening, I dine with everyone else."

"Our guest is really coming for that thing called time," says Deborah. "Most of us don't have enough of it in our lives, to sit in bed in the morning and think, or walk up a mountain. We allow a woman to decide what she wants to do, and we enable her to look with pride on what she has accomplished during the week, so she'll feel more competent in selecting a challenging life when she leaves."

This night those on the liquid diet sit separately from the others, since the aroma of eggplant parmesan can be very unsettling when one is drinking broth and munching seeds. You notice that dishes are smaller than normal so it looks like you're getting more. How clever! You vow to do the same—using demitasse spoons and cocktail forks—when you return home.

DAY 3

This begins like an ordinary day, but it's not. It's your midweek weigh-in, and there is a lot of speculation about it. Good news—you're down two pounds. You relax. After weigh-in the day proceeds pretty much like the previous ones: breakfast in your room. Your thimbleful of bran, seeds, and raisins mixed with apple juice is followed by a baked egg in a pretty cup with a quarter of a slice of toasted homemade bread wrapped in gold foil. You eat very slowly, recalling Deborah's words from the previous evening's talk. "You have to become aware of what you're putting in your body. You move 10 percent less for every decade of life, so you have to eat less. But the quality of the food becomes more important because it still has to do the whole job, or more of a job. Visualize the energy in the food you eat; double your pleasure by eating slowly." Suddenly less feels like much more. You start counting. The egg takes twenty bites to finish. You stretch that minute morsel of bread to ten bites. It can be done, but you have to concentrate.

You're ready for warm-up exercises. Your schedule is similar to day 1, but the activities are a little more strenuous as you become accustomed to doing them. The instructors have changed, and each new one brings with her special tricks and techniques. This third day, though, is a difficult one—a turning point, say those who have come before. You feel sore, tired, hungry, and your body grudgingly adjusts to all the beneficial things you're doing for it. You may feel a bit low psychologically as well, but you're assured of feeling better tomorrow. You hope you will.

Lunch at poolside. You're sitting next to a woman who recently spent a week at another spa. She didn't lose a pound but loved the beauty program. This is her second week at the Door. She vows to stay as long as it takes to lose all the weight she wants to. You wonder whether it's possible to incorporate the Door's tenets when you're back in the city. You remember three of Deborah's tips that make perfect sense, and promise to try them:

• realize that the average restaurant plans its portions for an active man five feet ten inches tall, so that you, since you're smaller, gain weight. In fact, any time you take in more calories than you expend, your body stores them as fuel. If you do eat out often, learn to like ethnic foods of people small in stature—Japanese, Chinese. Portions are usually smaller.

• shop daily. In this way you can buy the freshest produce in the exact amount you need.

• serve food directly from the

kitchen and avoid big platters in the center of the table. Portions can then be scaled to your size.

Many of the guests continue Virtue-making Day at home once a week, usually on Mondays. All agree that they have in some way changed their eating habits since their first spa stay. One woman has a rather expensive solution to portion control in a restaurant—but her slim form shows it works: She has the waiter remove half of everything from her plate. Another drinks only wine spritzers, for half the calories, or alternates a glass of wine with one of Perrier. Another snacks on raw vegetables before she goes to a restaurant, so that she won't eat everything in sight once she gets there. You decide that since dessert is your favorite part of the meal and you can't live without it, you'll start sharing it. In that way you'll still have your taste of something sweet, but at a fraction of the calories. If you save just 100 calories a day, you'll lose ten pounds over the year!

DAY 6

The day of truth. You're weighed and measured after your morning walk and learn that you've lost 5 pounds and a total of ten inches from those thirteen body spots. Best, two of those inches are off your waist and one inch is off each of your thighs. Today you feel good—and that news makes the day even better.

Last evening's cooking class was decidedly one of the highlights of your stay—you learned how to make the dishes you liked most, plus how to decalorize those you normally make. Chef Michel cooks with practically no oil, lots of fresh herbs, and thickens his sauces with Neufchâtel cheese. Portions of fish and chicken are small—about 3½ to 4 ounces—and salads are large; he mixes salad dressings thin so that they coat the greens, then fall to the bottom of the dish and stay there, instead of on your hips. His delicious potassium broth seems easy to duplicate—to a tomato and shallot base you add whatever vegetables you have in the refrigerator, simmer all for forty-five minutes, strain, and serve garnished with hot pepper flakes. "I made it at home last year, but it didn't taste the same," complains one woman. "Perhaps it was because the total ambience of this place was missing." Certainly food is a preoccupation here. You remember that the most animated conversations at the dinner table concerned restaurants and recipes. Dinner, though, has been remarkably pleasant. This group has been a very friendly one, which of course has helped contribute to everyone's good time.

Classes are more intense this day. "Lower that leg, ladies. Hold it back," screams your instructress. "Slower, slower, do you all know what 'restraint' means?" she asks. "If we did, we wouldn't be here," quips a voice in the rear.

You meet with your fitness advisor to make a tape of those exercises you need most, so that you'll do them at home. Aerobics are essential after forty to increase and maintain cardiac reserve. Spot exercises, too, tighten those flabby areas—you want to try to do them daily. Your exercises are set to music exactly as they are in class.

Yesterday you had a jazz dance session with Yuichi, a noted choreographer. Today it's tap-dancing, replete with bow tie, tap shoes, and cane—top hat, too. Next, your massage—you're no longer sore. After having your hair washed and styled, you dress for dinner. Tonight is graduation, and the change in everyone is miraculous. Faces glow, and it's not just from makeup. The effects of a hard and steady workout have made all the difference. You sip a champagne glass of white wine or Perrier, or a spritzer, in celebration of the weight-loss and inch-loss winners—at 8½ pounds, and 17¼ inches respectively. One of them is the woman who had gained 40 pounds. The total group lost 127¼ pounds—"We lost a whole person," remarks someone. Total inches lost, a high 328. The winner of the "pool," at 326, receives a handsome mirror. After dinner you are presented with your diploma, a perfect ending.

DEPARTURE

This mornings's activities include a walk, breakfast, then abbreviated exercise sessions. You're leaving before brunch, so a box lunch has been prepared. Your bag is packed, the car is waiting to take you to the airport. You take one last look at your slimmer silhouette, at the smooth-fitting trousers that seven days ago were uncomfortably snug. As you're leaving, one of the women mentions that she thought breakfast was almost too large. She actually left a few demitasse spoonfuls of bran and barely finished her egg topped with mushrooms and cheese, and half slice of toast with honey. "I was really stuffed. Do you think I'm learning portion control?" You cross your fingers and hope that you, too, having learned the golden mean, can keep sight of it when your spa experience is just a happy memory!

SELECTING THE SPA FOR YOU

Naturally, your spa experience depends upon the spa you visit. Some spas concentrate on weight control, others on beauty services. Some are renowned for their food, others are less gourmet. Weather, price, and size of the group should also influence your choice. Go about choosing a spa carefully. Send or call for brochures, and don't hesitate to ask questions. The following spas have excellent reputations and may provide you with just the experience you've been searching for (all prices are approximate, and may be subject to a service charge—usually 15 percent—and sales tax):

Golden Door, P.O. Box 1567, Escondido, California 92025. (714) 744-5777. Approximately $2,275 per week.

The Greenhouse, P.O. Box 1144, Arlington, Texas 76010. (817) 640-4000. Approximately $2,200 per week.

Owned by two experts on women—Neiman-Marcus and Charles of the Ritz—The Greenhouse is another ultra-posh beauty haven. The beauty-grooming program is particularly outstanding—every possible service is provided. Each guest even receives a tray of cosmetics and colors to experiment with. Balanced with the two to three hours of beauty each day are approximately five hours of exercise designed to reshape and retone the body. Diet is an important part of the overall program, and menus are built around 850 calories. The rooms are airy and charming, the entire setting, in fact, a flowering greenhouse, as the name suggests. Accommodations are for thirty-eight women. Leotards, tights, jogging suits, and bathrobes are provided, but you wear your own clothing for dinner.

Maine Chance, Phoenix, Arizona 85018. (602) 947-6365. Approximately $2,000 per week.

This well-known beauty retreat was created by Elizabeth Arden on a lush 105 acres, verdant with palm trees, cactus, groves of orange and lemon trees, and gardens of floral blossoms, overlooking the famous Camelback Mountain. The feeling here is of being in a private home, lovingly furnished and art-filled. Emphasis is on beauty and grooming—massage, steam, sauna, Ardena wax baths and whirlpool, daily face, hair, and nail treatments, as well as makeup classes. The ninety minutes of daily exercise are divided into three thirty-minute sessions; the routines were developed by the famous expert Marjorie Craig. The low-calorie diet is nutritious and filling and based on 900 calories. Accommodations are for fifty guests, dress is casual, and exercise clothes are provided, but you do have to bring your own clothing to wear for dinner. Evening activities include theater trips in Phoenix, movies, games, and television.

The Phoenix, 111 North Post Oak Lane, Houston, Texas 77024. (713) 680-1601. Approximately $2,150 per week.

This elegant spa is set like a tiny jewel in the vast Houstonian complex—which contains a private club plus hotel (spa guests stay in a private section of it), a health and fitness center, a productivity and a preventive medicine center—of eighteen wooded acres surrounded by a jogging path. Dedicated to offering each guest a lifetime plan of cardiovascular health, exercise is emphasized heavily, but a multitude of beauty services are offered as well—manicure, pedicure, facials, waxing, hair care and styling, and a daily massage. All manner of exercise classes, presided over by Director Chris Silkwood, formerly with the Golden Door, are available in the carpeted exercise rooms located in the landmark Art Deco House and in the graceful adjoining pool. In addition, guests have full use of the Houstonian's racquetball and tennis courts, running track, equipped gyms, volleyball courts, and outdoor Olympic-size pool. The food is deliciously low-calorie—850 calories unless you are there to gain weight—and beautifully presented. Accommodations are for thirteen women, and all clothing—except leotards, tights, and shoes—including caftans for evening, is provided.

Rancho La Puerta, Tecate, California 92080. (714) 478-5341. Plans for three, five, or seven days. On a weekly basis, least expensive accommodation is $750 per person for a cabaña. (If two persons share a room, the rate is $600 per person.)

A rustic hideaway on the Baja Peninsula, Rancho La Puerta was founded by Deborah Szekely eighteen years before the Golden Door. Here, health and fitness are key and pampering is at a minimum—the facials and massage are top-notch, though. Expect hikes and vigorous walks and the Fitness Parcours, a two-mile stretch of track interspersed with twenty exercise stations—each with directions and equipment for a specific exercise. Food is mostly vegetarian and calorie-controlled at 1,000 calories. The atmosphere is low-key but high-energy. Facilities are co-ed, and there are approximately 125 guests at any one time.

The following three spas are associated with hotels/resorts—guests have the option of enrolling in the spa program. All have separate facilities for men and women. Spa guests can mingle freely with non-spa guests at mealtimes and any other times they are not engaged in activities.

Gurney's Inn, Montauk, Long Island, New York 11954. (516) 668-2345. The seven-day plan costs approximately $450 plus the room rate, which begins at $74 per person, double occupancy. Shorter-stay plans are available.

All services here have an international influence. Interesting skin and body treatments include the Salt-glo loofah rub, Thalasso therapy (water-jet massage), Italian Fango Packs (hot mud), herbal and kelp wraps, and French Vichy sessions, as well as the Russian steam rooms and Finnish saunas. The setting—a luxurious inn with a commanding view of the ocean—is superb, as is the giant indoor seawater pool. Exercise sessions are continuous and include a fitness program for executives. Complete beauty services are available, as is a low-calorie meal plan worked out in advance with the spa nutritionist. Approximately twenty full-time spa guests go through the program at any one time. Only robes and slippers are provided.

The Spa at the La Costa Hotel and Country Club, Del Mar Road, Carlsbad, California 92008. (714) 438-9111. Minimum of four nights, approximately $225 per day single, and $335 double.

At any hour of the day you might see at least three celebrities around the pool at La Costa—some of the hundred guests that go through the spa each day. The experts here feel it is important that spa guests learn control in the surroundings that make up their life-style, so they are not isolated from temptations. You can be served your low-calorie meal in any of four dining rooms. Your spa program is designed after a consultation with a spa counselor; activities include a daily massage, facial, and makeup class, plus at least two exercise sessions. You also receive the obvious beauty services—manicure, pedicure, herbal wraps, and hair care and styling. Special services are available at an added charge. Exercise clothing is provided, but you do dress for dinner. Evening activities are arranged for spa guests, but there are always ongoing movies, dancing, and backgammon.

The Spa at Palm Aire, 2601 Palm Aire Drive North, Pompano Beach, Florida 33060. (305) 972-3300. Florida residents: (800) 327-4960, toll-free. Seven-day plan approximately $1,685 for a single-occupancy accommodation and $2,650 for a double. A four-day plan is also available.

The Spa at Palm Aire is part of a 1,500-acre resort/recreation community with five golf courses and thirty-seven tennis courts. The basic seven-day Renaissance plan begins with a medical examination and consultation, then includes a daily gymnastics class, yoga, jogging, water exercises, and Parcours exercise routine, daily massage, facial, herbal wrap, whirlpool, Swiss shower, alternate-day Salt-glo loofah scrub, plus steam, sauna, beauty services at the Spa salon, and classes in self-discipline, weight control, and behavior modification. A Spa sports program consisting of regular Spa activities in the morning and golf, tennis, and sports in the afternoon, as well as an executive fitness program, are also offered. Low-calorie meals are offered in the Spa's dining room, and you are free in the evenings to shop at the nearby plaza or enjoy the area's entertainment if you do not want to engage in the evening spa activity. Accommodations are for ninety women; robes, slippers, and warm-up and exercise clothing are provided.

Chapter 17

Fifty Tricks That Put Time on Your Side

1. Keep your expression "enigmatic," counsels Dr. Norman Orentreich. Exaggerated facial expressions—grimaces, broad smiles, squinting—lead to wrinkles and deep lines, while a placid one (look how smooth the Mona Lisa's face seems) prevents their occurrence.

2. Facial exercises, too, put a strain on your skin, continues Dr. Orentreich, and only aggravate facial-expression grooving. If you want to tone the muscles in the lower part of the face, he suggests raising and pressing the back of your tongue to the roof of your mouth.

3. Skin that's lined, no matter how slightly, looks less so if it's dampened, then moisturized.

4. No product you can buy removes wrinkles, contrary to any cosmetic claim made. However, there are temporary tighteners on the market that smooth skin for a few hours. You can make your own undereye tightener by beating the white of an egg until foamy, then painting a thin film under the eyes with a brush. When it dries, pat your foundation lightly over the area. This smooth film can crack, though, from the movement of your facial expressions.

5. Insure your skin's lifetime good looks by adjusting your treatment products to its seasonal needs: when skin is dry, stay away from strong detergent soaps and anything alcohol-based; when it's oily, avoid cleansing creams and lotions—they're too rich and heavy.

6. Remember, too, that skin is different all over your face, so you'll need a combination of products. And they don't have to come from the same company to do the job—mix and match products for the best results.

7. How effective are the products you use? If they make you feel better, you'll probably look better. The brain affects the skin's behavior in ways that are still not fully understood.

8. As epidermal turnover time slows down, cellular debris builds up. Don't add to it by sleeping with your makeup on. Always cleanse your face thoroughly before you sleep.

9. Circulation lags with the years, so that we slowly lose facial rosiness. Stimulate the blood flow and bring color back to your cheeks without exercising by relaxing on a slant board for ten minutes a day.

10. A more mature complexion shows exhaustion faster than a younger one and looks even older as a result. Whenever you're tired, get an instant glow by exercising for

several minutes before applying your makeup.

11. Stimulate facial color with a mask; mix yogurt with honey and smooth over clean skin. Leave on for fifteen minutes, then rinse off with tepid water.

12. You're never too old for break-outs and blemishes. Treat isolated trouble spots with an acne preparation containing benzoyl peroxide. For any condition more severe, consult your dermatologist.

13. For many women after forty, dry skin is really a problem. If you like the refreshing action of a toner (particularly cooling in hot weather) but find even an alcohol-free one too harsh, try patting it on with a *damp* cotton pad.

14. Lined skin looks older, feels more uncomfortable after a day outdoors in the blustery cold. Ease irritation and dryness with this soothing tip from free-lance expert Gary Bowers: Cleanse your face with cream, then smooth on petroleum jelly and step into the bath or shower. The heat will help the jelly penetrate. After your bath, tissue off excess and, if you're applying makeup, sweep a toner-saturated cotton pad lightly over your skin to remove any greasy residue.

15. Even though most complexions become drier over the years, there are those that become oilier. Papaya juice cuts down on shine and sluffs skin gently. Pat it over your face, wait five minutes, then rinse off with tepid water.

16. Stay younger-looking longer by staying out of the sun. And those times when you are exposed, protect your skin all over with a sun-screen that contains benzophenone, not just para-aminobenzoic acid (PABA), because it screens out both types of ultraviolet rays—A as well as B; PABA screens out UVB rays only. While UVB is the primary source of sun damage, UVA not only deepens the melanin deposits already found in the skin (darkening freckles) but has recently been found to act as a UVB enhancer as well.

17. It's never too late to try something new—like tinted contact lenses. You might find that changing or intensifying your eye color gives your look a wonderful kick. But don't forget to adjust your makeup and wardrobe shades accordingly.

18. Tired eyes add years. Keep yours bright without the aid of drops by placing your index fingers at outer eye corners and pressing gently for a minute or two.

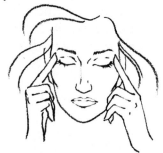

19. Another eye soother, good for reducing puffiness as well: cucumber slices! Lie down with your head

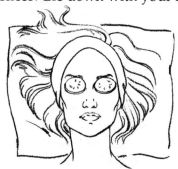

raised slightly and put thin slices of cucumber over your closed eyelids for fifteen minutes.

20. Beauty expert Shelley Durham points out that you should color-compensate for pigment changes in your hair and skin after forty. He suggests assembling color swatches from a paint store and holding them against your skin while you look in a mirror. You can then easily judge which shades do the most for you!

21. Let your surroundings as well complement your coloring. Create a flattering backdrop by decorating your home in the colors that suit you best, make you feel best.

22. Night light can be draining—you need flush and glow when it gets dark. Here's where a makeup mirror with different light selections makes mistakes impossible.

23. After forty especially, a very shiny face is not seductive, says makeup artist Pablo. Keep shine to a minimum with *light* dusting of powder.

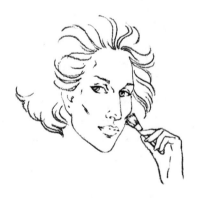

24. Too many facial angles might be too much of a good thing. Fill in cheek hollows by powdering them lightly with a pale ivory face powder. Finish your face with a hue that matches your skin more closely.

25. The single biggest beauty mistake the after-forty-year-old makes, agree the experts, is to do too much—or nothing at all! Check your look and make the necessary adjustments.

26. "One focal point is all the forty-year-old face can carry," says beauty authority Stan Place. So, if your mouth is bright red, shade the rest of your face neutral and low-key. Decide where your strength is, then play it up.

27. Don't wear bright blue or green eye shadow on your lids—too harsh and artificial. Leave them to the very, very young, if anyone.

28. Aging: skintight chignons—they emphasize lines and wrinkles; long straight hair—it drags features down. Speak to your hair stylist about a hairdo with lift and bounce. Ask, too, what a gentle body permanent can do for your hair.

29. If your tresses are brittle and lifeless, blame your hair-care habits rather than your age. You might not be rinsing out your shampoo thoroughly. Try washing your hair in the shower, avoiding rubbing and tugging, then condition regularly until your hair is back in shape.

30. Both age and the environment take their toll on hair now, when thickness counts most. Your hair is most voluminous when it's clean, but even conditioner can weigh it down. If you need conditioner, apply a *small* amount to hair ends only, and rinse out thoroughly.

31. Stress levels are often at an increase now—and that can lead to hair fallout. Trichologist Philip Kingsley advises eating mushrooms if you have this problem, since he

believes that they inhibit the chemical processes taking place in the body causing hair to fall out in the first place.

32. Deprivation can lead to tension—and tension shows in your face. So reward yourself. Whether it be a beautiful sweater to show off your slimmer figure, or even a chunk of chocolate because you've been dieting all week (you can compensate for it tomorrow)—you deserve it!

33. Offset any thickening through your middle by simply standing tall. Good posture slims your waist instantly and counteracts any aging slouch. Moreover, your spine will be more efficient, and any pressure on your nerves will be released.

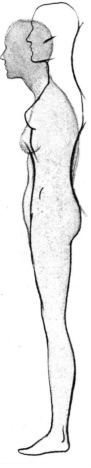

34. If you're not shaping up quickly enough, you may be expecting too much too soon. It takes more than a month of exercise for every year of inactivity to get your body back in form.

35. Every calorie counts—so don't rest between exercises, because when you do, the number of calories you burn per minute drops by 50 percent or more.

36. And calories are used differently at breakfast than at dinner. Studies into the body's daily rhythms indicate that you can lose weight or gain weight from the same meal—depending on the time of the day you eat it: it's less fattening in the morning than at night.

37. Taking control of your life now can really give you a feeling of power—a strong antidote to helplessness and depression. Start by taking control of your weight—keep a diary to pinpoint habits that need changing. Every day note what you eat, the time you ate, how long it took to eat, your mood at the time, the serving size, calories, with whom you ate and where. Use this information to tailor a diet plan just for you.

38. Your goal—to lower calorie-intake and increase calorie-expenditure: studies show that you'll stay with a diet and an exercise plan longer if you're part of a group.

39. How can you make less taste like more? By including nutritious foods that fill you fast, thus cutting your appetite—like whole grain breads and baked potatoes. Whole grain bread provides fiber, among other essentials, while a medium-sized baked potato contains only 145 cal-

ories packed with protein, carbohydrates, vitamin C, iron, thiamine, riboflavin, niacin, and very little fat.

40. Another way to reduce calories without trying: eliminate 3 teaspoons of sugar a day from your coffee and you'll lose about 4½ pounds a year.

41. A too-quick, too-drastic weight loss can make you look haggard and drawn—your skin's fat pads help keep it firm and rounded. The safe way to jolt off 5 pounds fast, though, is to halve your food portions while doubling your exercise.

42. Don't "up" your sodium intake, particularly if you are postmenopausal, but do drink lots of water. However, some carbonated mineral waters have a high sodium count, even though you can't taste the salt. Check to see that yours is salt-free.

43. Painful leg cramps, often more frequent with age, result from lack of exercise and improperly fitting shoes. Strengthen your calf muscles by standing on a telephone book with your heels hanging over the edge. Let them drop to the floor,

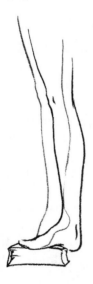

then raise up on your toes. Repeat ten to fifteen times a day. Make sure that new shoes fit by trying them on at the end of the day when your feet are slightly swollen. (If cramps are due to varicose veins, check with your doctor.)

44. Your hands need exercise as much as the rest of you, for muscle tone and bone density. Squeeze a soft rubber ball with your fingers five times daily, then stretch arms out to the sides and rotate wrists slowly in a clockwise direction five times, then counterclockwise five times.

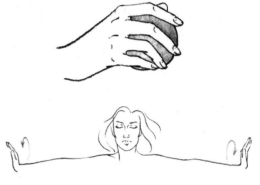

45. Since nails grow more slowly through the years, give them all the ammunition they need to stay supple, so breaks and cracks are at a minimum. Every week, soak them—without polish—in warm oil (any kind will do) mixed with several drops of lemon juice (a natural whitener) for twenty minutes.

46. Never wear eyeglasses on a chain or charm bracelets—they date you!

47. Ditto for necklaces with your first name on them. Select classic shapes in real or real-looking gold or gems. Appearing rich never goes out of style.

48. The right earrings after forty are

important; they can visually "correct" a thinning or drooping lower face. Wear bulky (outsized, too, if you're tall) geometric shapes for width.

49. Dangling earrings are usually difficult to wear now because they can "pull" your face down. Counteract this by styling your hair up and off your face and choosing earrings with width and body, plus length.

50. After fifty, alcohol can actually improve your health—in moderation, that is. Research indicates that it boosts the formation of HDL or "good" cholesterol—the kind that protects against heart disease—which otherwise decreases after menopause.

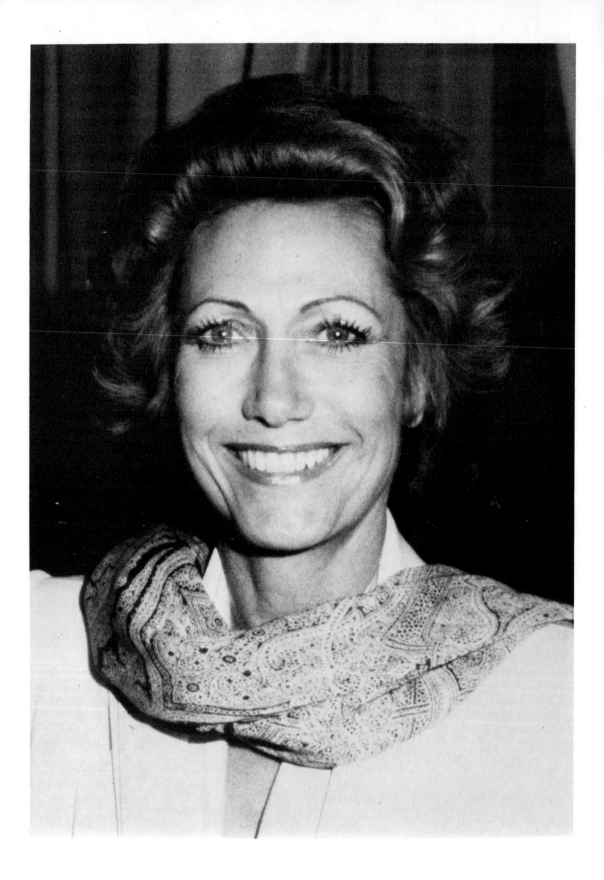

Hélène Rochas

*Creative advisor and spokeswoman,
Parfums Rochas, Paris*

*You're in your flower in your twenties—it's the springtime. Between thirty
and forty, it's summer. After forty, it's autumn, but that's also a good season.
The leaves are falling, but there's beauty, too. What you have inside counts
most. The best makeup is what you project, and I think Lena Horne exemplifies
this perfectly. She's suffered, but the experience has made her very interesting.*

*I was eighteen years old when I met my husband. He told me I was not
chic—because young women never are. Of course, times were different then,
but a woman doesn't learn who she is until she has experience. When you are
young, you haven't suffered, and you're not such a perfectionist. Now you've
done it all, and you probably know what happiness means. You feel that you
need time—each moment is very important. The more you know, the more you
know you don't know. Experience makes us strong, but we're also weak, and
fragile. Afraid, perhaps, maybe not as free as we think. Women live in a sort
of second youth after forty. But our complexes are different from the young. I
used to be very anxious when I was young, but I no longer am. The best part
of my life has been after forty. The young are free and very self-absorbed. At
my age we live for love and friendship; we know what friendship means.*

*I think the most important thing is love. A man who is my life. That's how
a woman stays feminine, by loving and being loved. But she has to be ready
to give something, too. Chanel once said, "Men love women not because they
are strong, but because they are weak." After forty, we are strong in business
but not in love. We're very insecure; that's why we're appealing. But of course
that depends upon the woman, too. In France, men are more open to women
who are past forty. You often see an older woman with a younger man. Maybe
he wants to learn. Of course, at the beach young women look good—their
bodies are better. But during the evening the woman over forty looks more
glamorous and elegant.*

*When I met my husband, I was studying to be an actress, but he did not
want me to continue. He was a designer, and when we married, created a
perfume for me, called Femme. I was thirty when he died, and continued as
president of his company, which was very successful. I created the fragrance
Madame Rochas. Then I sold Parfums Rochas, but ten years later returned to
it as creative advisor and spokesperson. I'm involved in all art and creation.*

Art has always been a great love of mine, and I've long been friendly with people in the arts.

Perfume is naturally a very important part of my life—it's the music of the heart. I think all women need perfume. It's an attitude, and should be the last thing she puts on before going out. Because life is stronger now, fashion, too, perfume is as well. I change scents, alternate them. At the moment I like a more flowery fragrance. I don't know why. Perhaps we're entering a period of florals.

My skin has changed, but it's never been delicate. Usually it's normal, but in New York I find that it is much drier. I cleanse it with soap, use a little freshener, and rinse with Evian water. I use an eye cream and a light moisturizer, then a sheer foundation. I never sleep with a night cream. My makeup has not changed very much. I wear little. For evening I put more on my eyes and lips. In the country and on holidays I don't wear anything except mascara. I do sunbathe, but tan only my body—a little too much sometimes—not my face.

I've never had plastic surgery. The thought of it makes me uneasy. I like a face that is marked by life. Plastic surgery can be like a mask, unnatural. I've seen some terrible work. But many women feel they will be better afterward—it's often like seeing a psychiatrist. If you really need it, why not! I just don't think it's right for me.

My weight has stayed the same, but there are changes in my body. One always puts on inches where one doesn't want them. I walk and swim and do yoga. Anything that elongates the body is good. I eat a little of everything, but in very small amounts. I've always eaten very little. Some protein in the morning—yogurt with honey—then a very light lunch. At six I snack on cheese or ham to keep me from getting tired, since I dine very late. I eat a light dinner. I drink a lot of mineral water and tea, a little wine, and I don't smoke.

I'm always traveling, and have been all over the world. I know every country except China and India. When you travel, you learn. I like everything in life—art, music, books—I've been like this my entire life. You never get—or feel—old if you keep your curiosity; you're always learning. I have friends in their eighties who have not stopped being curious—they're happy.

I believe that beauty is a gift in life, but it's not enough. You have to be rich inside. There are so many women with a beautiful face and figure who are lost because they are lazy. But many times the woman who is not so beautiful is the greatest success because she works hard to be something.

Index